Sustainable
Diets, Food, and Nutrition

PROCEEDINGS OF A WORKSHOP

Leslie Pray, *Rapporteur*

Food Forum

Food and Nutrition Board

Health and Medicine Division

The National Academies of
SCIENCES · ENGINEERING · MEDICINE

THE NATIONAL ACADEMIES PRESS
Washington, DC
www.nap.edu

THE NATIONAL ACADEMIES PRESS 500 Fifth Street, NW Washington, DC 20001

This activity was supported by contracts between the National Academy of Sciences and the National Institutes of Health (HHSN263201200074I/HHSN26300079); the U.S. Department of Agriculture (59-8040-7-001, AG-3A94-C-17-0009, USDA-CNPP-FF-17-DC, and USDA-OFS-NAS-17-DC-01); and the U.S. Food and Drug Administration (HHSP233201400020B/HHSP23337012), with additional support by the American Heart Association; Cargill, Inc.; Chobani, LLC; The Coca-Cola Company; Conagra Brands; General Mills, Inc.; Keurig Dr Pepper; Mars, Inc.; Nestlé Corporate Affairs; Ocean Spray Cranberries, Inc.; PepsiCo; and Unilever. Any opinions, findings, conclusions, or recommendations expressed in this publication do not necessarily reflect the views of any organization or agency that provided support for the project.

International Standard Book Number-13: 978-0-309-47955-4
International Standard Book Number-10: 0-309-47955-X
Digital Object Identifier: https://doi.org/10.17226/25192

Additional copies of this publication are available from the National Academies Press, 500 Fifth Street, NW, Keck 360, Washington, DC 20001; (800) 624-6242 or (202) 334-3313; http://www.nap.edu.

Printed in the United States of America

Suggested citation: National Academies of Sciences, Engineering, and Medicine. 2019. *Sustainable diets, food, and nutrition: Proceedings of a workshop*. Washington, DC: The National Academies Press. doi: https://doi.org/10.17226/25192.

The National Academies of

SCIENCES • ENGINEERING • MEDICINE

The **National Academy of Sciences** was established in 1863 by an Act of Congress, signed by President Lincoln, as a private, nongovernmental institution to advise the nation on issues related to science and technology. Members are elected by their peers for outstanding contributions to research. Dr. Marcia McNutt is president.

The **National Academy of Engineering** was established in 1964 under the charter of the National Academy of Sciences to bring the practices of engineering to advising the nation. Members are elected by their peers for extraordinary contributions to engineering. Dr. C. D. Mote, Jr., is president.

The **National Academy of Medicine** (formerly the Institute of Medicine) was established in 1970 under the charter of the National Academy of Sciences to advise the nation on medical and health issues. Members are elected by their peers for distinguished contributions to medicine and health. Dr. Victor J. Dzau is president.

The three Academies work together as the **National Academies of Sciences, Engineering, and Medicine** to provide independent, objective analysis and advice to the nation and conduct other activities to solve complex problems and inform public policy decisions. The National Academies also encourage education and research, recognize outstanding contributions to knowledge, and increase public understanding in matters of science, engineering, and medicine.

Learn more about the National Academies of Sciences, Engineering, and Medicine at **www.nationalacademies.org.**

In memory of
Leslie A. Pray
1964–2018

PLANNING COMMITTEE FOR A WORKSHOP ON SUSTAINABLE DIETS, FOOD, AND NUTRITION[1]

CONNIE AVRAMIS, Research and Development Director, Nutrition and Health, Unilever

ADAM DREWNOWSKI, Professor of Epidemiology and Director, Nutritional Sciences Program, School of Public Health, University of Washington

JESSICA FANZO, Bloomberg Distinguished Associate Professor, Global Food and Agriculture Policy and Ethics, Nitze School of Advanced International Health, Bloomberg School of Public Health, Johns Hopkins University

KATE J. HOUSTON, Director, Federal Government, Relations/Corporate Affairs, Cargill, Inc.

PAMELA STARKE-REED, Deputy Administrator, Nutrition, Food Safety, and Quality, Agricultural Research Service, U.S. Department of Agriculture

PARKE E. WILDE, Professor, Friedman School of Nutrition Science and Policy, Tufts University

---

[1]The National Academies of Sciences, Engineering, and Medicine's planning committees are solely responsible for organizing the workshop, identifying topics, and choosing speakers. The responsibility for the published Proceedings of a Workshop rests with the workshop rapporteur and the institution.

FOOD FORUM (AS OF AUGUST 2018)[1]

[1]The National Academies of Sciences, Engineering, and Medicine's forums and roundtables do not issue, review, or approve individual documents. The responsibility for the published Proceedings of a Workshop rests with the workshop rapporteur and the institution.

KRISTIN REIMERS, Conagra Brands, Omaha, Nebraska
CLAUDIA S. RIEDT, Keurig Dr Pepper, Plano, Texas
SHARON A. ROSS, Division of Cancer Prevention, National Cancer Institute, National Institutes of Health, Bethesda, Maryland
PAMELA STARKE-REED, Agricultural Research Service, U.S. Department of Agriculture, Beltsville, Maryland
REGINA L. TAN, Office of Food Safety, Food and Nutrition Service, U.S. Department of Agriculture, Alexandria, Virginia
DOROTHEA K. VAFIADIS, American Heart Association, Washington, DC
JEFFREY J. ZACHWIEJA, PepsiCo, Barrington, Illinois

Health and Medicine Division Staff

HEATHER DEL VALLE COOK, Food Forum Director
ROMY NATHAN, Program Officer
ANNA BURY, Research Associate (*through August 2018*)
SYLARA MARIE CRUZ, Research Associate
CYPRESS LYNX, Senior Program Assistant
ANN L. YAKTINE, Director, Food and Nutrition Board

Reviewers

This Proceedings of a Workshop was reviewed in draft form by individuals chosen for their diverse perspectives and technical expertise. The purpose of this independent review is to provide candid and critical comments that will assist the National Academies of Sciences, Engineering, and Medicine in making each published proceedings as sound as possible and to ensure that it meets the institutional standards for quality, objectivity, evidence, and responsiveness to the charge. The review comments and draft manuscript remain confidential to protect the integrity of the process.

We thank the following individuals for their review of this proceedings:

NAOMI K. FUKAGAWA, U.S. Department of Agriculture
KATE J. HOUSTON, Cargill, Inc.
HELEN H. JENSEN, Iowa State University
PARKE E. WILDE, Tufts University

Although the reviewers listed above provided many constructive comments and suggestions, they were not asked to endorse the content of the proceedings, nor did they see the final draft before its release. The review of this proceedings was overseen by **HUGH H. TILSON,** University of North Carolina. He was responsible for making certain that an independent examination of this proceedings was carried out in accordance with standards of the National Academies and that all review comments were carefully considered. Responsibility for the final content rests entirely with the rapporteur and the National Academies.

Contents

1

Introduction

The banana is a staple of U.S. households and the world's most exported fruit. Yet, it is difficult to produce and ship bananas while simultaneously protecting the environment from degradation and promoting fair economic practices to benefit all stakeholders. Thus, the banana exemplifies the complex, multidimensional challenges to achieving sustainable diets, stated Sylvia Rowe, SR Strategy, LLC, Washington, DC, and chair of the Food Forum of the National Academies of Sciences, Engineering, and Medicine, in her opening remarks at the Food Forum's workshop on Sustainable Diets, Food, and Nutrition held in Washington, DC, on August 1 and 2, 2018. Moving forward, Rowe asserted, if the banana is to retain its favored fruit status, its agricultural practices will need to be transformed and equity promoted throughout its supply chain.

These and related challenges and the opportunities for addressing them were the subject of the workshop (the Statement of Task for the workshop is highlighted in Box 1-1).[1] According to Rowe, one of the strengths of the Food Forum is its ability to find concordance and synergy by bringing people from different disciplines and sectors together. She expressed the hope that the presentations, discussions, and even disagreements throughout the workshop would foster both ideas and multisector action.

[1]The planning committee's role was limited to planning the workshop, and this Proceedings of a Workshop was prepared by the workshop rapporteur as a factual summary of what occurred at the workshop. Statements, recommendations, and opinions expressed are those of individual presenters and participants, and are not necessarily endorsed or verified by the National Academies of Sciences, Engineering, and Medicine, nor should they be construed as reflecting any group consensus.

BOX 1-1
Workshop Statement of Task

An ad hoc committee will plan and convene a 1.5-day public workshop that will review the current and emerging knowledge on the concept of sustainable diets within the field of food and nutrition. Broadly, the workshop agenda will explore sustainable diets and relevant impacts for cross-sector partnerships, policy, and research. Workshop presenters may also discuss how sustainable diets could impact dietary patterns, the food system, and population and public health. The workshop could also address research gaps, advances in knowledge, and innovation.

The planning committee will define the specific topics to be addressed, develop the workshop agenda, and select and invite speakers and discussants. After the workshop, proceedings of a workshop—in brief and full proceedings of the presentations and discussions at the workshop will be prepared by a designated rapporteur.

The organization of this Proceedings of a Workshop parallels that of the workshop (see Appendix A for the workshop agenda). Chapter 2 explores the complexities and necessary compromises of sustainable diets (Session 1). Chapter 3 examines the challenges of and opportunities for measuring diet and modeling the human and environmental impacts of dietary and agricultural changes (Session 2). Chapter 4 describes what modeling and other studies suggest about program and policy actions that can support sustainable diets (Session 3). Building on the foundation laid in the earlier chapters, Chapter 5 further explores and adds new perspective on food system innovations designed to address sustainability (Session 4). Finally, Chapter 6 summarizes several participants' reflections on the workshop and their main takeaways (Session 5). All of the chapters conclude with summaries of the open discussions that took place at the end of each session.

2

What Are Sustainable Diets?

In the first session, moderated by Fergus Clydesdale, University of Massachusetts Amherst, speakers explored the complexities and necessary compromises of sustainable diets. This chapter summarizes the Session 1 presentations and the discussion that followed. Highlights of the presentations are provided in Box 2-1.

THE DIMENSIONS OF SUSTAINABILITY

Setting the stage for presentations to follow, Adam Drewnowski, University of Washington, Seattle, emphasized the multiple dimensions and interdisciplinary nature of sustainability. He called attention to two documents. He first described the 2005 Giessen declaration, which articulated the concepts of personal, population, and planetary health. He remarked that this was the first time he had seen mention of "personal, population, and planetary health" in a nutrition journal. The declaration, which, he asserted, should have received a wider audience, stated that the new nutrition science ought to encompass social, economic, and environmental as well as biological dimensions, and that the study of integrated food systems should serve as the basis for food and nutrition policies (Beauman et al., 2005). The document was signed by a number of prominent nutrition experts, he added, with the intent of embracing other sciences and clearing the way for a more interdisciplinary approach to nutrition. Drewnowski then called attention to the 2012 Food and Agriculture Organization (FAO) report *Sustainable Diets and Biodiversity* (FAO, 2012b). It was from this report

BOX 2-1
Highlights of Individual Presentations*

- The Food and Agriculture Organization's (FAO's) definition of a sustainable diet consists of four dimensions: (1) nutrition and health, (2) economic, (3) social and cultural, and (4) environmental. Sustainable diets not only have low environmental impact but also are healthy, affordable, and acceptable to society. (Drewnowski)
  - Because of these multiple dimensions, sustainable diets encompass inherent tensions and contradictions. (Drewnowski)
  - The trade-offs and compromises required as a result of these tensions and contradictions are context-specific. They vary regionally and among countries, but also among neighborhoods. (Drewnowski)
  - The development of models that can be used to predict future impacts of diet requires thinking about food systems, not just individual foods, and integrating data and metrics from multiple sources. (Drewnowksi)
- Sustainability in the context of diet is not a new issue. The challenge is how to turn today's more complex, nuanced definition of sustainability into a feasible reality. (Fanzo)
  - The challenge is particularly difficult for those living in low- and middle-income contexts and in countries where tremendous inequalities force policy makers to make difficult decisions about what to prioritize. (Fanzo)
  - Much of the challenge stems from the rapid demographic transition under way worldwide, with increasing wealth, urbanization, and other factors driving a growing demand for meat. (Fanzo)
  - Policy making is a messy, unpredictable process. To better integrate sustainability issues into policies relevant to diets and nutrition, scientists need to engage with the policy process as it exists. (Fanzo)
- A key challenge stemming from the multisectoral nature of sustainable diets is communication among the sectors. (Wilde)
  - Food prices are a form of communication. They are like the aperture on a camera: a price may seem like a small hole, but in fact, a great deal of information passes through it, including information about sustainability. (Wilde)
  - Conversations about sustainable diets play out differently in low-priced versus high-priced environments. For example, decisions about holding land aside from agricultural production are easier to make in a low-priced environment, whereas the economic incentive to prevent food waste is stronger in a high-priced environment. (Wilde)
  - Because of the fluctuating nature of food prices, a goal should be to focus on pursuing a sustainable-diet strategy that encompasses both abundance (low prices) and scarcity (high prices). (Wilde)

---

*These points were made by the individual workshop speakers identified above. They are not intended to reflect a consensus among workshop speakers.

that he, as well as several other workshop speakers, drew their definition of sustainable diets (see Box 2-2).

The Four Dimensions of Sustainability: Tensions and Contradictions, Trade-Offs, and Compromises

According to Drewnowski, the FAO definition of sustainable diets has four dimensions: (1) nutrition and health, (2) economic, (3) social and cultural, and (4) environmental. He emphasized that sustainable diets not only have low environmental impact but also are healthy, affordable, and acceptable to society. In his experience, when people talk about sustainable diets, they are often talking only about the impact of diets on the environment, and he stressed the importance of including all four dimensions in such discussions. "Diets are not healthy *and* sustainable," he said. "They are sustainable only if they are healthy to begin with." In addition, though often missing from the discussion, are the economic and social dimensions.

Drewnowski went on to assert that the dimensions of sustainability lead to inherent tensions and contradictions. For example, he elaborated, some energy-dense foods cost less per calorie and may have a lower impact on the environment relative to other, more nutritious foods, but also have low nutrient density. An extreme case is sugar. "If you want a plant food with the lowest land cost, lowest water use, and lowest greenhouse gas emissions," Drewnowski observed, "look no further than sugar."

Drewnowski explained that the trade-offs and compromises necessitated by these inherent tensions and contradictions call for a focus on food systems rather than individual foods. He added that all of the various connections along the food system path lead from production to consumption to waste and disposal (Downs et al., 2017; FAO, 2012b; Johnston et al., 2014). He emphasized that optimization of all of the different considerations

BOX 2-2
What Are Sustainable Diets?

"Sustainable diets are those diets with low environmental impacts which contribute to food and nutrition security and to healthy life for present and future generations. Sustainable diets are protective and respectful of biodiversity and ecosystems, culturally acceptable, accessible, economically fair and affordable; nutritionally adequate, safe and healthy; while optimizing natural and human resources."

SOURCE: FAO, 2012b (as presented by Adam Drewnowski).

that arise is context dependent as the trade-offs are not necessarily the same for all countries or regions, or even for all neighborhoods.

According to Drewnowski, modeling sustainable food systems and predicting and optimizing all of the various considerations involved requires gathering and integrating data from multiple sources, both private and public. He remarked that one of the intents of this workshop was to bring together experts familiar with these types of models and data sources. He noted, too, that this modeling is a two-way street: existing diets can affect the climate, which in turn can affect future diets. Because diets can be either the cause or the outcome, he observed, "to some extent, existing diets are paving the way for future diets."

The Metrics of Sustainable Diets

Drewnowski went on to explain that each of the four dimensions, or domains, of sustainable diets relies on a different set of measures and metrics. He then described some of these metrics.

Nutrition Domain

When assessing nutrition, two key measures Drewnowski uses in his own work are energy density (dietary energy per unit weight) and nutrient density (nutrients per reference amount). He remarked that the concept of nutrient density can be complex, and different ways of measuring the nutrient density of foods (e.g., using nutrients per calories or nutrients per unit weight for nutrient profiling) have been the subject of recent discussions. He explained that nutrient profiling is a technique for rating individual foods based on their nutrient content or ratio of nutrients to calories. Without going into detail, he mentioned the European Food Safety Authority (EFSA) guidelines for nutrient profiling and noted a current trend toward what he termed "hybrid nutrient profiling," whereby not just nutrients but also healthy food ingredients can contribute to an overall nutrient density score (Drewnowski and Fulgoni, 2008). In his opinion, measuring nutrient density in terms of nutrients per 100 kilocalories (kcal) is arguably more useful than measuring nutrients per 100 grams (g) or per serving. The former approach, he elaborated, allows for direct comparisons of affordability, generally measured as calories, or nutrients per unit cost. He added that measuring cost per calories makes it possible to see, for example, that energy-dense foods (fats, sugars, and grains) often have lower nutrient densities compared with vegetables and fruit (see Figure 2-1). He noted that energy-dense sweets and fats tend to cost less per calorie and may have a lower environmental footprint, but they also tend to be nutrient-poor. He noted that not only have energy-dense foods become dominant in the food

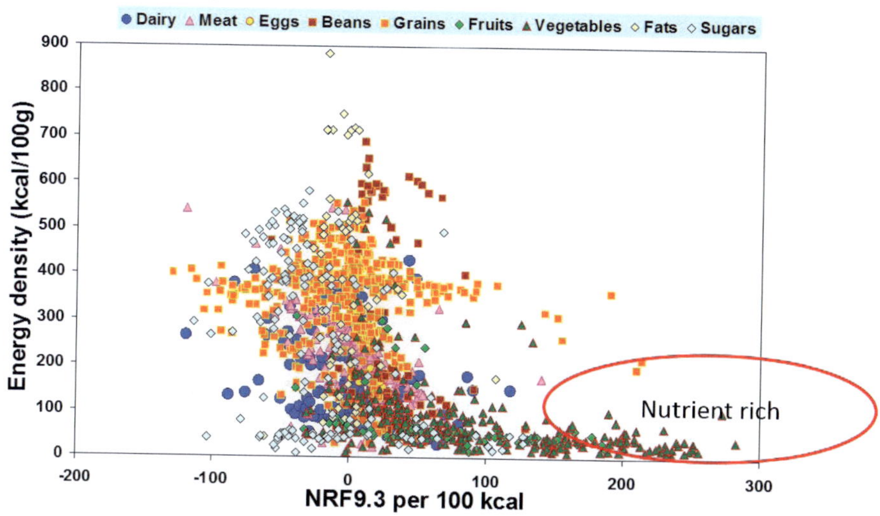

FIGURE 2-1 The relationship between nutrient-rich foods and energy density.
NOTES: NRF = nutrient-rich food. The y-axis depicts energy density as kilocalories (kcal) per 100 grams; the x-axis depicts nutrient-rich foods by NRF 9.3, which is a European Food Safety Authority nutrient profiling score.
SOURCES: Presented by Adam Drewnowski on August 1, 2018, from Drewnowski, 2017.

supply, but research suggests that high energy density promotes overeating and leads to overweight.

Drewnowski also pointed out that many energy-dense foods are plant foods. "We actually overconsume plant foods," he said, which include vegetable oils, sugars, and high-fructose corn syrup, adding that less energy-dense plant foods may be more satiating at fewer calories, but are also considerably more expensive in terms of per calorie monetary cost.

Economic Domain

Drewnowski went on to observe that the finding that nutrient-dense foods typically cost more (see Figure 2-2) has been noted not just in the United States, but also in France and Mexico. He suspects that the same is true in low- and middle-income countries as well.

Environmental Domain

According to Drewnowski, more nutrient-dense foods and more nutrient-dense diets also typically entail higher carbon costs. He remarked

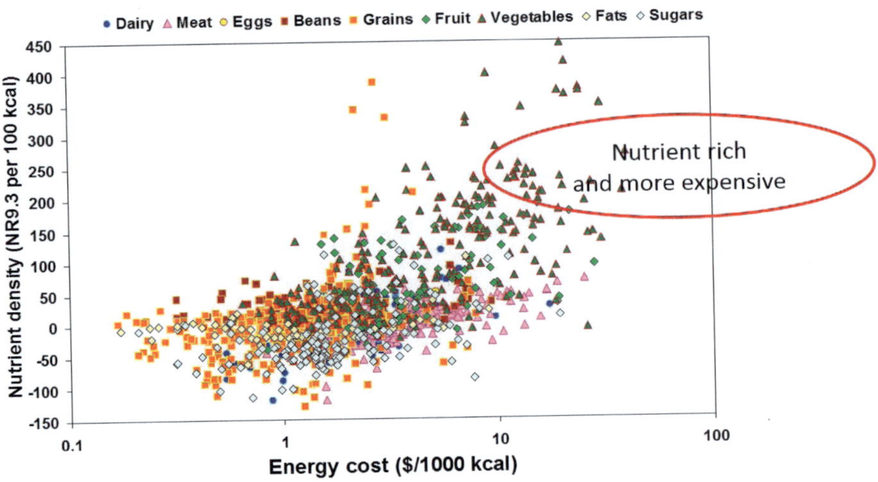

FIGURE 2-2 Relationship between monetary cost ("energy cost," or dollars per 1,000 kilocalories [kcal]) and nutrient density (NRF 9.3 per 100 kcal).
NOTES: NRF = nutrient-rich food. The y-axis depicts nutrient density by NRF 9.3, which is a European Food Safety Authority nutrient profiling score; the x-axis depicts energy cost as U.S. dollars per 1,000 kcal.
SOURCES: Presented by Adam Drewnowski on August 1, 2018, from Drewnowski, 2017.

that carbon cost is often calculated per 100 g or per kilogram of food with little attention to what the food actually is, and stated that he prefers to measure carbon cost from the standpoint of calories. Given that an individual needs 2,000 calories or a certain amount of protein per day, for example, one can then ask about the environmental cost of producing those calories or grams of protein. In Drewnowski's opinion, weight is entirely immaterial when one is comparing emissions of greenhouse gases (GHGs), given that some foods are mostly water (e.g., there is actually more water per gram in spinach than in a carbonated soft drink). In contrast, he continued, comparing GHG emissions based on calories reveals a direct linear relationship between the nutrient density of foods and their carbon costs per 100 kcal (see Figure 2-3). "Nutrient-rich foods actually are more costly from the standpoint of energy than are candy and sugar," he pointed out, adding that there is also a linear relationship between total dietary calories and GHG emissions. "The more calories people eat," he said, "the more carbon energy the diets consume."

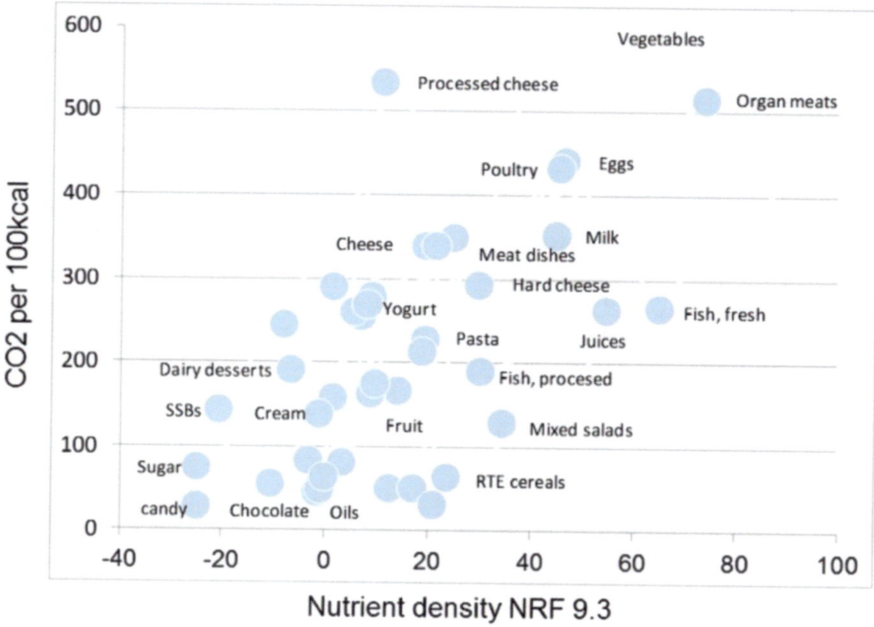

FIGURE 2-3 The linear relationship between nutrient density and carbon cost.
NOTES: CO_2 = carbon dioxide; NRF = nutrient-rich food; RTE = ready-to-eat; SSB = sugar-sweetened beverage. The y-axis depicts carbon cost as CO_2 per 100 kilocalories (kcal); the x-axis depicts nutrient density by NRF 9.3, which is a European Food Safety Authority nutrient profiling score.
SOURCE: Presented by Adam Drewnowski on August 1, 2018.

Social Domain

In the social domain, Drewnowski called for measuring food patterns rather than individual foods or nutrients when assessing the relationship between diet and health outcomes, especially obesity. Food patterns are determined by society more so than the consumption of individual nutrients or foods, he asserted. Yet, he observed, studies in nutrition epidemiology typically link individual nutrients, foods, or dietary ingredients with health outcomes while failing to adjust for socioeconomic status, past history, culture, and other contextual factors. To illustrate this point, he described how in Seattle, a map of the consumption of soda by neighborhood showing that people living in less expensive houses near freeways consume more soda relative to people living in mansions on the waterfront costing several million dollars can be overlaid on a map of the distribution of obesity by neighborhood. The comparison reveals more obesity near the freeway than on the waterfront. Thus, Drewnowski argued, improving the healthy eating index among people living in neighborhoods near the freeway "is not simply a question of getting people to switch from one food to another ... it is all about geography, education, income, and food patterns."

Final Remarks

Ending on what he termed a provocative note, Drewnowski suggested that researchers studying obesity replace their focus on individual dietary components with a focus on food patterns. He pointed to different studies on obesity, both by the same researchers and both published in the same journal but several years apart, with one implicating dietary fat (Bray and Popkin, 1998) and the other high-fructose corn syrup (Bray et al., 2004). "I think that we need a paradigm shift," he argued.

In closing, Drewnowski called for multiple types of input data, assessments of the costs and benefits of alternative diets, estimates of likely regional compromises and trade-offs, and models that are sensitive to prices and social concerns. Finally, he emphasized the collective nature of the endeavor to achieve sustainable diets and urged the engagement of academia, governments, nongovernmental organizations (NGOs), and the food industry.

IMPLICATIONS AND RELEVANCE OF SUSTAINABLE DIETS INTERNATIONALLY: IT'S ALL ABOUT THE CONTEXT

Building on Drewnowski's presentation while also placing evidence on sustainable diets in a political context, Jessica Fanzo, Johns Hopkins University, Baltimore, Maryland, began by talking briefly about what she described as the "long, tangled history" of discussions around sustainable diets. Today, she noted, sustainable diets are being discussed in global reports, such as the 2016 report of the Global Panel on Agriculture and Food Systems for Nutrition, *Food Systems and Diets: Facing the Challenges of the 21st Century* (GLOPAN, 2016); the *Global Nutrition Report 2017* (Development Initiatives, 2017); and the 2017 report of the Committee on World Food Security, *Nutrition and Food Systems* (HLPE, 2017). But, she observed, the topic is not new: "It comes in and out of fashion," she said. She mentioned Joan Dye Gussow's work on ecological nutrition in the 1970s and Gussow's book *Chicken Little, Tomato Sauce, and Agriculture: Who Will Produce Tomorrow's Food?* (Gussow, 1991). She agreed with Drewnowski, however, that past discussions centered mainly on the environment and human health, with little consideration of economic, sociocultural, and other factors that are recognized today as being so important to sustainable diets.

Turning the Food and Agriculture Organization (FAO) Definition of Sustainable Diets into a Feasible Reality

Fanzo characterized the goal of turning the 2012 FAO definition of sustainable diets (see Box 2-2) into a feasible reality as a "real challenge," particularly for those living in low- and middle-income countries and in contexts where tremendous inequalities force policy makers to make difficult decisions about trade-offs. Consumers, too, must navigate sustainable diets, she added. Currently, she observed, it is difficult to understand what foods are and are not sustainable, and what to believe and not believe about what is written about food and diets in the media. She added that consumers also must consider taste, preference, convenience, practicality, and affordability to fulfill their own demands and desires. The private sector, in turn, must answer to those demands while ensuring that there is a market for its products and that consumers have economic incentives to buy them. In sum, Fanzo said, many stakeholders must be considered when determining how to turn the definition of sustainable diets into a reality.

Sustainable Diets in Low- Versus Middle- Versus High-Income Countries

Fanzo went on to state that in some low-income contexts, where populations cannot necessarily afford animal-sourced foods, many of the diets consumed are plant-based and could be considered quite sustainable in the way they are grown and processed. She pointed to a working paper by the World Resources Institute showing global differences in daily protein consumption (based on supply chain data). According to that paper, daily per capita protein consumption is lowest in India and highest in Brazil, followed by the United States and Canada (Ranganathan et al., 2016). As urbanization and economic growth progress, Fanzo observed, meat consumption is rising, with some exceptions.

The question then arises of whether the plant-based diets consumed in many low-income contexts are sustainable, Fanzo continued, and whether they are fulfilling the nutritional needs of those communities. Animal-sourced foods are important for growth, she noted, particularly for young children. She characterized as controversial the conclusion in a recently published paper in *Lancet Global Health* that in sub-Saharan Africa, particularly in west Africa, people are eating among the healthiest diets in the world (Imamura et al., 2015), given that malnutrition burdens (stunting, micronutrient deficiencies) remain high in that region. She added that, based on an analysis of 2016 UNICEF global data, children aged 6 to 23 months worldwide are eating one type of animal-sourced food per day or none at all. In many places, she reported, even if young children are eating a diet diverse in plant-based foods, with many legumes and leafy greens, they still lack access to enough iron and zinc in their diet, as illustrated by data from Bangladesh, Ethiopia, and Vietnam (Dewey and Vitta, 2013). Iron and zinc, she emphasized, are critical micronutrients for cognition and growth.

Regarding climate change, Fanzo observed, an additional challenge for low-income countries is that they are affected by the dietary decisions of those living in higher-income countries. "Our choices about what we consume will impact those people who have the inability to adapt and deal with climate change," she said. "Our choices matter."

Global Transitions and Transformations: The Growing Demand for Meat

Expanding on the observations summarized above, Fanzo explained that the world is undergoing rapid demographic, epidemiologic, and nutrition transitions: urbanization is expanding, with people moving from rural, subsistence-agriculture landscapes into urban centers; people have more disposable income; physical activity is changing; the food system is becoming increasingly global; and health outcomes also are changing, as seen in rising rates of obesity and diet-related noncommunicable diseases. Although approximately 1 billion people go to bed hungry every night, while another billion are purposely exercising and consuming a healthy diet, most of the world—about 5 billion people—is in a state of rapid transition, including rapid shifts in diet (Crino et al., 2015; Drewnowski and Popkin, 2009; Fanzo et al., 2017). Fanzo herself spends a great deal of time in Myanmar, where, she said, the "hippest" restaurant at present is KFC. Why? "It taps into desire," she explained, recalling queues five blocks long to get into a KFC in Yangon. Of this growing demand for meat, she said, "I cannot emphasize that enough," adding that it is not just the demand for meat that is growing worldwide (see Figure 2-4), but also the demand for animal feed. "This whole system needs to be rethought," she argued, stating that those 5 billion people are less able to access what would be considered a healthy, sustainable diet today than they were in the past.

Disjointed Policies and Policy Trade-Offs

Dietary guidelines are almost always a mismatch with what agricultural systems and the food supply can bear, Fanzo continued, because food-based dietary guidelines are often developed without the involvement of agronomists and environmental scientists. To illustrate this point, she cited work by Steven Wiggins at the Overseas Development Institute (ODI) who has demonstrated that if everyone followed the U.S. *Dietary Guidelines for Americans* (DGA), the world's dairy supply would be outstripped (Wiggins and Keats, 2014). Other research has shown that agriculture systems are

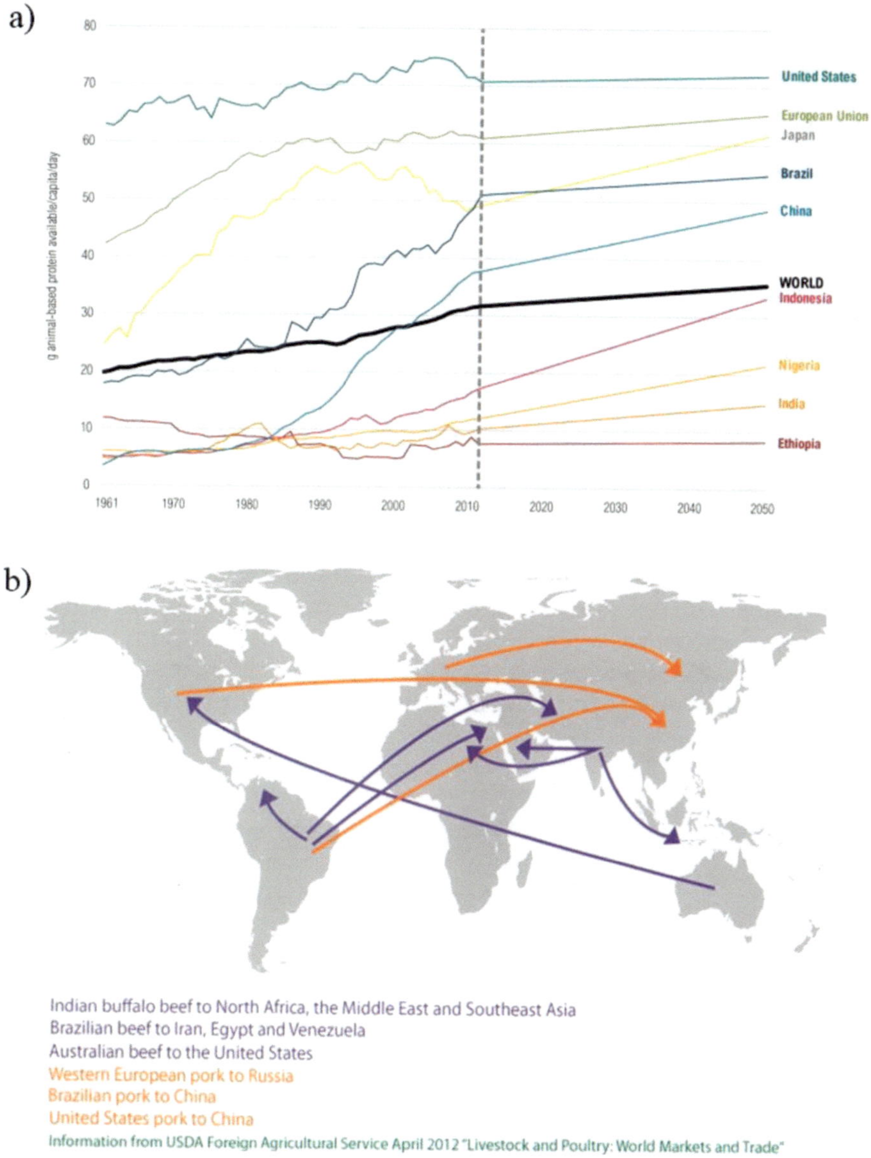

FIGURE 2-4 The growing demand for meat: (a) daily animal-based protein availability per capita (i.e., based on supply chain data), 1961–2050; (b) examples of the movement of meat globally.
SOURCES: Presented by Jessica Fanzo on August 1, 2018, modified from Ranganathan et al., 2016.

becoming more homogeneous, she added, with fewer crop species responding to a growing demand (Khoury et al., 2014). Again, she urged greater thought as to what agriculture can deliver toward the achievement of nutritional goals. She stressed that policy makers are constantly dealing with these trade-offs, citing environmental, health, and economic trade-offs involved with such commodities as palm oil, olive oil, and grassfed beef, to name a few.

Trade policies play a part as well, Fanzo continued. She and her colleagues, for example, recently published a study showing an increase in the number of people with micronutrient deficiencies in the absence of trade (Wood et al., 2018). "There are always these trade-offs that we have to consider," she reiterated.

Evidence Gaps

Fanzo agreed with Drewnowski that there are clear gaps in scientists' understanding of what constitutes a sustainable diet for different populations and how sustainable diets in different contexts are best measured. More specifically, she called for better characterization of the key determinants of a sustainable diet and how these determinants can be measured in a spatiotemporal way, using a suite of indicators such as those described by Drewnowski. In addition, she called for guidance on what a sustainable diet would mean economically for all actors in the food value chain, particularly in low- and middle-income countries. For example, if industry is being asked to become more sustainable, what does that mean for this sector economically?

Finally, Fanzo called for policy analysis to better integrate sustainability issues into policies relevant to diets and nutrition and to create what she described as "policy coherence." She mentioned a recent study in which she and her colleagues examined a suite of indicators and then plotted them on different countries to create "dashboards" (Gustafson et al., 2016). But, she asked, would a policy maker sitting at his desk in Senegal and looking at this dashboard diagram know what to do with it? "Probably not," she said, acknowledging that she was critiquing her own work, and explaining that policy makers are thinking more about value chains and how to "get food from A to B to C" (Fanzo et al., 2017). The question for them, she elaborated, is how to inject sustainability into a value chain. Thus, instead of handing policy makers a suite of indicators or a dashboard and telling them to look at the data, she stressed, "we need to start thinking like policy makers and understanding what they need to make an informed, evidence-based decision."

In another recent study, Fanzo and colleagues examined three different national strategies in Nepal: the Multi-Sectoral Nutrition Plan, the National

Biodiversity Strategy and Action Plan, and the Agriculture Development Strategy. They systematically examined whether the three strategies captured elements of sustainability across a range of themes, including environmental, sociocultural, economic, and nutritional. Their results showed that the Agriculture Development Strategy included the most sustainability elements, and the Multi-Sectoral Nutrition Plan the least (Downs et al., 2017). "What does this say?" Fanzo asked. "We need to get the global nutrition community thinking about sustainability," she suggested. Agriculture thinks about it more, she said, because it is their "bread and butter."

Coming to Grips with Evidence-Based Policy Realities

While the hope is that all policy making is rooted in solid evidence, Fanzo continued, in reality there is no policy-making cycle in which to inject evidence at the point of decision making (Pew-MacArthur Results First Initiative, 2014; Sutcliffe and Court, 2005; Young and Quinn, 2002). The policy-making cycle typically involves an assessment, then a budget, then implementation, followed by monitoring and readjustment, she elaborated, describing policy making as a messy, unpredictable, complex process. Evidence may resonate, or it may not, she explained. When policy makers are making decisions, she observed, they do look at evidence, but they also use judgment; gather information from lobbying groups; and consider their country's habits, traditions, and values. Thus, while evidence-based policy may be improving, policy is still also opinion based (Davies, 2004; Sutcliffe and Court, 2005). For researchers who work with evidence, Fanzo suggested, this can be a difficult reality to grasp. So while she agreed with Drewnowski that more evidence is needed, she believes researchers need to start thinking about what to do with that evidence. Policy makers do not read *Nature* or *The Lancet*, she observed, nor is writing a policy brief enough, in her experience. She spoke of the "bounded realities" within which policy makers are operating and their need to make quick decisions with limited information. In sum, she asserted, "we need to reject romantic notions that policy makers think like us, as scientists, and that there is an identified point of decision at which experts can contribute to the evidence that makes an impact."

In Fanzo's opinion, given how the world has rallied around the Sustainable Development Goals (SDGs), now is an opportune time to reinvigorate the dialogue on sustainable diets. She mentioned that all United Nations (UN) Member States would be meeting in 2019 to report on where they are with respect to the SDGs and identified that meeting as an important venue for examining what has been achieved in the area of sustainable diets.

In closing, Fanzo cited an article that had just been published that morning (August 1, 2018) in *The New York Times* about how the science around climate change was clear enough three decades ago that it could be laid out well for policy makers, along with solutions for how to address it (Rich, 2018). But then, she said, concern about climate change went out of fashion. Now, she asserted, it is back in fashion. "This is my call to all of you," she stated, "that maybe we know enough. There has been a lot published on sustainable diets. We need to be thinking about ensuring that this kind of thing does not happen again, where we knew what to do 30 years ago, and policy makers just did not act on it." She ended by saying, "Be thinking policy."

DECISION MAKING UNDER UNCERTAINTY: SUSTAINABLE DIETS FOR CONDITIONS OF SCARCITY OR ABUNDANCE

Parke Wilde, Tufts University, Boston, Massachusetts, began by asserting that the inherently multisectoral nature of sustainable diets requires engaging, in the same forum, people thinking about public health and nutrition, about the environment and climate change, about food consumers, about supply chains and food waste, about farmers and food producers, and about reducing poverty (FAO, 2012b; Johnston et al., 2014). These people are not thinking the same thoughts, he observed, nor do they share the same goals. Controversy ensues, he explained, whether the topic is dietary guidelines, food labeling, carbon taxes, farm subsidies, genetically modified organisms (GMOs), agricultural conservation programs, water allocation, or something else. Thus, he argued, sustainable diets are contentious, and the question then is how these sectors can talk to each other.

Wilde offered several suggestions for communication among the various sectors, beginning with workshops such as this and documents such as *Sustainable Diets and Biodiversity* (FAO, 2012b) and the recently released *Sustainable Diets* (Mason and Lang, 2017). Eco-labels and other food labels are another forum for communication, he added, explaining that food labels not only reach greater numbers of people relative to workshops and documents, but also are valuable for linking information across different stages of the food marketing chain. But, he noted, labels have shortcomings based on a complexity that requires considering a number of different factors to ensure that consumers can make use of the labels. As another forum for communication, Wilde cited the production standard checklists (e.g., standards for safety or ecology) that are negotiated between agricultural producers and input suppliers on the one hand and food retailers, buyers, or the intermediaries who represent them on the other. Although less visible than labels to the public, these checklists are contentious, highly negotiated documents specifying what the standards of production should be.

Food Prices as a Forum for Communication

Wilde then turned to a final forum for cross-sector communication—prices. It is widely thought that prices are too thin a signal to be useful for this purpose, he remarked. However, he observed, economists think of them as highly robust signals of what is going on in different parts of the economy. He likened food prices to the aperture on a camera: it seems like a small hole, but in fact, a great deal of information passes through it. He asserted that food prices reveal much information about sustainable diets, such as what the demand is for different products under different conditions and what revenue farm owners and operators receive, how much farm laborers earn, how much healthy food costs for consumers, and what the big picture looks like with respect to scarcity and abundance. For the remainder of his talk, Wilde focused on the latter.

More specifically, Wilde described as the thesis of his talk that "conversations about sustainable diets play out differently in low-priced environments [abundance] and in high-priced environments [scarcity]. We need to be braced for both." For example, when food prices are low, conversations and public policy making around land conservation, such as whether to hold land aside from agricultural production, are easier to conduct than is the case in a high-priced food environment. As examples of such conversations, Wilde cited decisions that need to be made with respect to the U.S. Department of Agriculture's (USDA's) Conservation Reserve Program or, in Malaysia, about palm oil, mentioned earlier by Fanzo. On the other hand, he observed, some conversations are easier when food prices are high, including conversations about livelihoods for farmers, economic incentives to reduce food waste, and investments in alternatives to traditional meat products.

The Economics of Sustainable Diets: How Cost Is Passed Down the Market Chain

Wilde argued that if economics are part of a sustainable diet, with all stakeholders earning a reasonable livelihood, it is essential to understand how cost can be passed down the marketing chain. A photograph that he took of a Coalition of Immokalee Workers (CIW) rally for better wages in March 2018 showed dozens of protestors on a street, all wearing coats; some wearing winter caps; and many holding signs, including two people holding a banner reading "Fighting for Fair Food! Luchando por Comida Justa!" The question, he said, is not why these people are rallying for better wages or a better piece rate on the tomatoes they harvest—"That stands to reason," he said—but why they are wearing winter coats and why they are rallying in New York City in March rather than in Florida. The answer, he said, is prices. He explained that tomato growers in Florida are in a competitive business in which they can claim, with complete credibility, that it is very difficult for them to agree to higher wages because competitive pressures prevent them from passing that cost down the food marketing chain. In contrast, he noted, the large companies that use tomatoes in fast food or retail chains are better able to absorb a higher wage. In this example, in Wilde's opinion, CIW's decision to focus on downstream buyers was a "very clever, wise, astute decision."

The History of Food Prices

Over the past six decades, food prices have risen and fallen, Wilde continued. The oil price crisis in the 1970s, he observed, along with weather and other production problems during that period, led to a sharp price spike. More recently, prices spiked again in 2008 and 2011.

Focusing on the past 30 years, Wilde described an initial long period of productivity growth in agriculture and trade that was associated with a fairly low price environment (from 1990 through the early 2000s) (see Figure 2-5). "People forgot to worry any longer about scarcity," he said. Two things then occurred as a result of changes in the agricultural economy, including increased use of food stocks for biofuels (in the early 2000s), which essentially removed those stocks from the human food supply. First, Wilde elaborated, prices started rising; second, prices fluctuated chaotically.

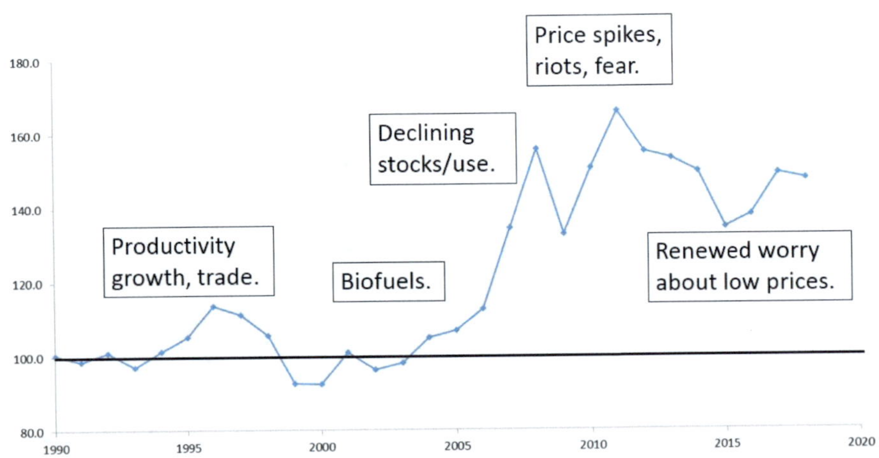

FIGURE 2-5 Food and Agriculture Organization (FAO) food price indices over the past 30 years.
NOTE: The y-axis depicts the FAO food price index; the x-axis depicts the year.
SOURCE: Presented by Parke Wilde on August 1, 2018.

He explained that changes in abundance from one year to the next are smoothed out as long as there is enough agricultural stock in the system. But without enough agricultural stock in the system, after several years in a row of low harvest and high demand, the stocks continue to decrease until they hit a point when they can no longer adjust smoothly from year to year, causing sudden price spikes. This, Wilde added, is what occurred in 2008 and 2011 (CFR, 2013). He recounted how both of those price spikes were associated with riots in developing country capitals and a great deal of fear around the world. After such price spikes, he continued, when prices fall again, as they did in the mid-2010s, people again start worrying about overproduction, excessive abundance, low prices, and how difficult it is for farmers to earn adequate livelihoods. Wilde cautioned, "We need to be worried about both types of conditions: high prices and low prices."

Thoughts on the Future of Food Prices

Wilde went on to note that USDA produces official projections of the future of food prices and other agricultural variables under certain assumptions. The projections for key row crops (soybeans, wheat, corn) through 2027, he reported, are neither as low as prices were in the 1990s or 2000s nor as high as the price spikes of 2008 and 2011. Nor do USDA's projected prices fluctuate as they have in the past decade. Similarly, Wilde continued, projected livestock prices through 2027, including those for beef cattle, broilers, and hogs, are somewhere in the middle. He explained that meat prices depend a great deal on how much is consumed, and while chicken consumption in the United States has been rising significantly in recent decades, USDA is forecasting a modulation of this increase. He added that consumption of both beef and pork has been declining somewhat and is expected to hold steady (USDA, 2018). In sum, he said, USDA is not predicting any radical change in where Americans get their protein, but is expecting more of the same. "That might or might not be the case," he observed.

Of the USDA price projections in general, Wilde said, "Not everybody agrees with this reasonably rosy view." He cited several assumptions underlying the projections. The first is mid-range economic growth in the United States (2.1 percent) and fairly good economic growth in developing countries (3.7–4.6 percent). Another assumption is moderate population growth (<1 percent globally, 1.1 percent in developing countries), which Wilde said is to be expected only if developing countries experience no economic collapse, women and girls continue to be educated at higher rates, and other social changes proceed well. As yet another assumption, Wilde cited moderate increases in energy prices (up to $80/barrel of oil), which he cautioned does not account for how climate change may impact the status quo. He noted that the USDA document containing these projections mentions neither climate nor warming, and it mentions drought only once, in an explanation of how future events and assumption variables are not certain. Additional assumptions, he reported, are no change in agricultural policy, although farm payments may rise; an initial increase in use of biofuels, but then a fallback; and current trade agreements remaining in place (USDA, 2018).

Wilde recounted how he reviewed a 2015 book, *The End of Plenty*, by Joel Bourne, Jr., which tells of the author's visits to farms in the Ukraine, places where fish are harvested in the middle of the Pacific, and elsewhere (Wilde, 2015). As a result of these trips, Wilde said, Bourne became very concerned about the future of abundance. In his book, the economist Malthus is a major figure. At the end of the book, the writer describes his trip to Bath Abbey in the United Kingdom to look for Malthus's gravesite. But he could not find it, Wilde said, and discovered later that the grave is hidden under the abbey's pews. The lesson, Wilde quipped, is that Malthus is "not yet ready to be resurrected." He warned, again, that while it is important to think about the possibility of price rises, it is also important to think about the possibility of overproduction and low prices that will threaten farmers' livelihoods.

Food Prices and Resilience

People need to focus not just on wishing for low prices, Wilde concluded, but also on the fundamental goals one hopes to achieve through low prices—namely environmental quality, healthy eating, a thriving economy, and low hunger and poverty. "Let prices be prices," he urged. "Let them do what they do well," which is to clear demand and supply quantities. He called for pursuing a sustainable diet strategy that does not assume just one future, but accounts for conditions of both scarcity and abundance.

DISCUSSION

Following Wilde's presentation, he, Drewnowski, and Fanzo participated in an open question-and-answer period with the audience, summarized here.

The Role of Technology

Earlier in the session, while introducing the speakers, Clydesdale had mentioned Sylvia Rowe's singling out of the banana as an exemplar of the challenges to achieving a sustainable diet (see Chapter 1). He had suggested that GMO technology may be the only way to deal with some of the sustainability issues related to the banana supply chain, raising both technological and social challenges. At the end of the session, he noted that there had been very little mention of technology during the presentations. He asked about the role of technology in what he described as "communities of plenty" versus "communities without plenty." He was curious about the role of technology in production, but also postharvest.

In response, Wilde commented on the importance of productivity growth and its major role in the low price environment of the 1990s and 2000s, even in the face of the opposition to GMOs and other new technologies. He said he suspects that some of this opposition will ease over the next few years as products come to market for the first time that are more visibly useful from a consumer perspective.

Fanzo agreed with Wilde that there is a role for technology in the agriculture sector and added that there is also a role for technology in shopping for and purchasing food. In China, for example, many 18- to 25-year-olds use an app on their smartphone to buy their food, which is delivered to their house cooked and ready to eat (CNBC, 2017). Even in the United States—in Seattle, for instance—Amazon is using "walk-in, walk-out" technology, much like that of driverless cars, in its new grocery stores. Instead of purchasing their food in checkout lines in which they engage with actual people, Fanzo elaborated, consumers take the foods they want to purchase off the shelves and walk out of the store without pulling out a credit card or money or even scanning the products. Purchases are all tracked through the consumer's phone. This technology raises "huge sustainability issues," Fanzo argued, including employment issues and issues around waste from prepackaged foods.

Drewnowski also agreed with Wilde that technology plays major roles in production, either by increasing yields or through fortification, but cautioned that more production does not necessarily lead to greater food security and public health. "There are all kinds of steps in between," he said. For example, he noted, more rice production does not solve the malnutrition problem in Southeast Asia. From a consumption perspective, he views technology as playing a role in helping to ensure a nutrient-rich diet for everyone, either through the reformulation of processed foods or perhaps through the fortification or biofortification of foods.

Finally, Clydesdale observed that technology has a role in dealing with waste as well.

How Policy Makers Make Decisions

There was some discussion in response to Fanzo's description of the way policy makers make decisions. Barbara Schneeman, University of California, Davis, expressed appreciation for Fanzo's description of that process and agreed that scientists need to think about how they fit into this paradigm. In her experience, science is necessary, but not sufficient; economic and legal elements are needed as well to create the political will to take meaningful action.

Denise Eblen, USDA, remarked that she always worries when someone says the science exists, and the challenge is to translate that science into policies. She mentioned how, in her past work at the National Institute of Food and Agriculture, increased production of food always drew greater interest than food safety or nutrition and was viewed as the biggest "bang for the buck." She asked how she, as a policy maker, can persuade other policy makers that it is not enough to produce food; rather, food must also be available, socially acceptable, and so on so that in 20 years, she is not looking back and thinking, "If only we had done that back then."

Drewnowski saw a connection to prices. There was a time when eating more calories meant getting more nutrients, he observed, but that time has passed, and today, people can eat extra calories without getting more nutrients, particularly if they are eating cheap foods. The connection between calories and nutrients is completely price-dependent now, he added. He encouraged USDA to update and revise the National Food Prices Database, noting that its last revision was in 2004. Having an updated database would be extremely helpful, in his opinion, as it would allow researchers to examine what it costs to have a healthy diet.

Wilde reframed Eblen's question: How does one communicate effectively and persuasively to policy makers and diverse constituencies to get them to understand the range of considerations that affect the same issues? "I have been stumped by that one so long," he said, "and have absolutely no answer."

Fanzo stressed, as she had during her presentation, that while much remains to be learned about sustainable diets, time is limited with respect to climate change. "We need to act now," she said. "We need to think about the evidence we have now."

Trade-Offs

With respect to the trade-offs and compromises entailed in sustainable diets, Schneeman asked, "If I can't have it all, what do I have to give up?"

Drewnowski replied that the role of modeling is to reveal the necessary compromises, or what the "sweet spot" is. He suggested that it is probably context dependent, with the right diet for one population being different from the right diet elsewhere. He mentioned recently having been in Southeast Asia as part of a study on nutrition transition and observing that people's choice of meat protein is highly dependent on culture, religion, and geography. He related that in one focus group, a man from Sulawesi,

Indonesia, said his family had been eating rice and fish for the past 30 years. To some people, that sounds like sushi, Drewnowski said, and they might think it was wonderful. But then the man's eyes started tearing up, and he said that he wanted to be able to give his family something that he could not afford, like chicken. "Aspirations and desires are very different," Drewnowski said. "We should not take them for granted."

From the perspective of a policy maker, for whom "it is all about making it to the next election cycle," Fanzo suggested that the "sweet spot" is short-term things they know will resonate with the people they prioritize. The question then is whether climate change is "one of those things that resonates? Is it visceral enough for people?" On the other hand, Schneeman pointed out that not all policy makers are elected officials; many are career staff.

Food Waste

If one believes that 40 percent of food is being wasted, Food Forum member Erik Olson, Natural Resources Defense Council, asked, "How is that issue being addressed in discussions on sustainable diets?" He commented on the enormous amount of wasted resources, such as cost, energy, and water, as well as emitted GHGs, embedded in all of that wasted food, and wondered why that had not been a prominent part of the session's discussion.

Wilde replied that he suspected that the 40 percent figure, as large as it is, refers to total food waste in the system. The more interesting figure for him is the estimate of economically recoverable food waste, that is, the amount of economically recoverable food that actually could be added back to the food supply. This amount changes, he said, depending on what is being used to save that food and on prices. He urged everyone to always read the "smaller number" (i.e., the amount of economically recoverable waste) in any report on food waste.

Human Health Costs and Other Externalities

While Olson said he was pleased that GHG costs are beginning to be integrated into conversations on the cost of food, as discussed by Drewnowski, he wonders how human health costs and other externalities besides GHG emissions are being addressed. For example, what about the costs to humanity of the obesity crisis? He asked whether there were any efforts to consider these other costs.

Drewnowski pointed out that the impact of diet on health would be addressed later in the workshop and that it is very much part of the modeling efforts around sustainable diets. With respect to other environmental costs besides that of carbon, he explained that it is difficult to obtain data on other aspects of the environment. Moreover, what data do exist often are region-specific. For example, data on water use from the Netherlands do not necessarily apply to southern California, and data on pasture in Switzerland do not necessarily apply to Australia. But Drewnowski agreed with Olson that other costs need to be considered. He called for a model that looks at the hidden costs of cheap diets in particular, while also noting that such costs cannot be separated from low wages, employment, and migration. Health is very much an outcome of food, he argued, but it cannot be linked entirely to the food choices people make. He underscored the importance of also looking at what drives food choices in the first place and referred again to the sharp social gradient of the obesity epidemic.

Cultural Shifts

For food companies to sell a more sustainable product, that product must be culturally relevant, Katya Hantel, Conagra Brands, remarked. "We have to attract consumers," she stressed. She added that in this regard, cultural relevance appears to be the most malleable criterion, especially in the current age of global connectivity. She pointed to insect flour as an example. In the United States, consumers can now purchase a protein bar that is made of insect flour, representing a shift in cultural appropriateness. She asked to what extent one can rely on what is culturally appropriate today, given such shifts. She also asked about the role of trying to shift what is culturally appropriate to encourage more sustainable diets.

Fanzo agreed that not only do trends shift, but different cultures tap into different trends. For example, she noted, today in the United States, sustainability is a trend, while in England, veganism is on the rise. She added that in many low- and middle-income contexts, what people tap into is more about achieving a better lifestyle and aspiring to become something, and food is a big part of that aspiration. She relayed what she had heard recently from someone in advertising: that people do not buy food because it is healthy or environmentally sustainable; rather, they buy food based on hope. "Why do we have Beyoncé advertising Pepsi?" Fanzo asked, replying because it taps into that desirability, that hope. In Kenya, she observed, fast food is not something people eat in their shambas—it is something they aspire to. "It is urban. It is modern. It is clean. It is safe," she said. In her opinion, that is what is driving cultural shifts.

The Effect of Greenhouse Gases on Nutrient Density

Maha Tahiri, former food industry executive, asked whether the effect of the current environment, specifically GHG emissions, on the nutrient density of food has been factored into the model Drewnowski had discussed (see Figure 2-3). Drewnowski replied that, although he had not factored this effect into that work, he had found in a recent study that GHG emissions, specifically CO_2 emissions under controlled conditions, reduced the nutrient content of rice (Smith and Myers, 2018). He agreed with Tahiri that the current environment will have an impact on the future nutrient density of foods.

3

Measurement and Analysis of Sustainable Diets from Production to Consumption

In Session 2, moderated by Diego Rose, Tulane University, New Orleans, Louisiana, speakers considered the challenges and opportunities entailed in measuring diet and measuring and modeling the human and environmental health impacts of dietary change and other sustainable diet strategies. Highlights of the presentations are provided in Box 3-1.

MAPPING FOOD SUPPLY AND DEMAND: DATA INPUTS, METRICS, AND MEASURES

Ashkan Afshin, Institute for Health Metrics and Evaluation (IHME), University of Washington, Seattle, provided an overview of the methods being used by the Global Burden of Disease (GBD) project to address common challenges to collecting and analyzing dietary data. Because the challenges are similar to those faced when analyzing health systems, he explained, much of what GBD researchers have been doing over the past decade is essentially applying lessons learned about the health system to the food system. Generally, he elaborated, they have been systematically identifying all relevant data sources and then harmonizing those data across the various sources and correcting for known biases, estimating all quantities of interest and the associated uncertainty and communicating the uncertainty level for each quantity to the public and policy makers, ensuring internal consistency in the data, and harnessing new data sources and new data processing methods to improve and update existing estimates.

BOX 3-1
Highlights of Individual Presentations*

- Although measuring diet poses a challenge, lessons learned from analyzing health systems are being applied. (Afshin)
  - There are many different sources of data on sustainable diets, and no single source is perfect. For example, food availability data are usually good in terms of coverage, but they do not reveal anything about consumption. (Afshin)
  - The Global Burden of Disease (GBD) project has combined and standardized multiple sources of data to characterize the human diet and estimate the burden of disease attributable to suboptimal dietary habits, a process that is updated annually. (Afshin)
  - Despite dietary data being far from optimal, multiple lines of evidence show that diet is an important risk factor for the health of people and the planet. (Afshin)
- Diet can be a major lever for addressing both human and environmental health. (Tilman)
  - If the current global dietary transition toward more calories, more meat, and more empty calories continues, greenhouse gas (GHG) emissions from global agriculture will increase substantially by 2050. If people were to adopt more plant-based diets, the increase in GHG emissions would be much smaller. (Tilman)
  - In addition to GHG emissions, food systems contribute to eutrophication (from fertilizer use and irrigation) and extinction (from land use). All of these environmental impacts have implications for the long-term sustainability of the support systems on which humanity depends. (Tilman)
  - The relationship between the human health and environmental impacts of foods is log-linear. Generally, foods that are healthy also offer great environmental benefits. (Tilman)
- The International Food Policy Research Institute's (IFPRI's) International Model for Policy Analysis of Agricultural Commodities and Trade (IMPACT) modeling system has been used to predict outcomes under different climate change, agricultural investment, and dietary shift scenarios. (Rosegrant)
  - Increased investment in agriculture can generate substantial increases in per capita income and reductions in hunger and stunting, water and land use, and GHG emissions. (Rosegrant)
  - Reducing per capita meat demand can reduce land loss, drive down meat prices, increase meat consumption in developing countries, reduce feed grain demand, reduce hunger, and reduce GHG emissions. (Rosegrant)
- Creating a resilient, sustainable food supply will require a balanced approach that entails both investing in agriculture and shifting diets toward less meat consumption. (Rosegrant)

*These points were made by the individual workshop speakers identified above. They are not intended to reflect a consensus among workshop speakers.

Comparing and Combining Dietary Data from Different Sources

According to Afshin, a key challenge with dietary data is that they are limited and scattered. Not all of the data are in the public domain, and what data are available are inconsistent across countries, as well as across sources within countries. Moreover, there are no links between agricultural and nutrition and health data. In other words, Afshin said, there is no food systems approach in the data collection.

The range of data on which GBD relies, Afshin continued, includes food availability data from the United Nations (UN) Food and Agriculture Organization (FAO), data on sales and purchases from Euromonitor, data on household expenditures on food from household budget surveys, dietary consumption data from both 24-hour dietary recalls and food frequency questionnaires, and biomarker data (e.g., to assess daily sodium intake). He observed that each of these types of data has both limitations and strengths. In fact, he said, one lesson IHME has learned over the years is that no single data source is perfect. To illustrate, he noted that food availability data have excellent coverage over time and across geography, but they do not reveal anything about consumption, such as age or sex patterns. On the other hand, dietary recall data are good in terms of providing data on age and sex patterns of consumption, but there is no good geographic representation of those data. And, Afshin added, there are limited nationally representative 24-hour dietary recall surveys that show trends over time. He explained that although sales data can be helpful for understanding consumption, they are generally not of good quality in low- and middle-income countries, they only help to understand recent trends in consumption, and reveal nothing about age or sex patterns. Finally, he noted, the limitation of biomarker data is that they are so sparse.

Again using lessons learned from health system analyses, Afshin reported, GBD researchers have been trying to combine these various sources of data, adjust for known biases, and make the data as comparable as possible. He explained how in past cycles of GBD, conventional statistical models were used to make the data comparable by first matching data by location, age group, sex, and time period, and then estimating relationships among the data in locations where there were enough data to do so and applying those relationships to other locations. More recently, he added, in the last round of GBD, the researchers tried some more advanced techniques involving machine learning and artificial intelligence to characterize relationships among the data. He noted that these novel methods significantly improved the estimation process. To illustrate, he described how the researchers modeled intake based on availability data by age, sex, and GBD super region (all countries are categorized into seven super regions, based on location), and then used those same data to train two different machine-learning methods to predict intakes based on data not yet seen and assess what is known as the out-of-sample predictive validity. He reported that for vegetable-related data, compared with an out-of-sample correlation of 0.45 for the conventional statistical model, both machine-learning methods significantly improved out-of-sample performance, with correlation coefficients of 0.95 and 0.92, respectively. The same performance comparison was carried out for all food groups included in GBD, as well as all nutrients. For many food groups or nutrients, the machine-learning models' out-of-sample correlations were around 0.80, Afshin said.

Afshin went on to explain that, after being made comparable, the data are combined to generate a single estimate of dietary consumption, again by age, sex, location, and year. This is done using a statistical method known as spatiotemporal Gaussian process regression to generate country-level estimates of intake (e.g., red meat in grams/day). Afshin added that this process is updated annually to include new data. He noted that, because high-quality consumption data were not available, the researchers' dietary estimates in earlier years (before 2000) were informed mainly by FAO food availability data and scattered data from household budget and dietary consumption surveys. In more recent years, however, their dietary intake estimates have been informed by more data from household budget and dietary consumption surveys. Again, Afshin noted, this single estimate, which represents the mean intake of each dietary factor, is generated for all dietary factors included in GBD by age, sex, location, and year.

Once this process has been carried out, Afshin continued, mean intakes in each country can be compared with recommended intakes. For example, as shown in Figure 3-1, fruit intake in much of the world is below the recommended level, whereas for the same sex and age group (males aged 45 to 49 in this example), red meat intake in many countries is above the recommended level. For nuts and fruits, Afshin reported, there is a huge gap at the global level between current consumption and recommended intake. The same is true of specific nutrients, such as omega-3 fatty acids, with the exception of Japan and other high-income Asia Pacific countries.

According to Afshin, in addition to comparing current and recommended intakes, GBD dietary data can be used to evaluate and answer other questions, such as how people replace different food items. For example, one of the most recommended replacements with respect to fatty acid intake is to replace saturated fat with polyunsaturated fat. In reality, however, people do not make that replacement, Afshin said; instead, they replace saturated fat with carbohydrates. Epidemiological evidence, he added, shows that saturated fat and carbohydrates are equally harmful.

Because not everyone consumes dietary factors at the mean level, Afshin continued, the next step is to estimate the distribution of usual intake for

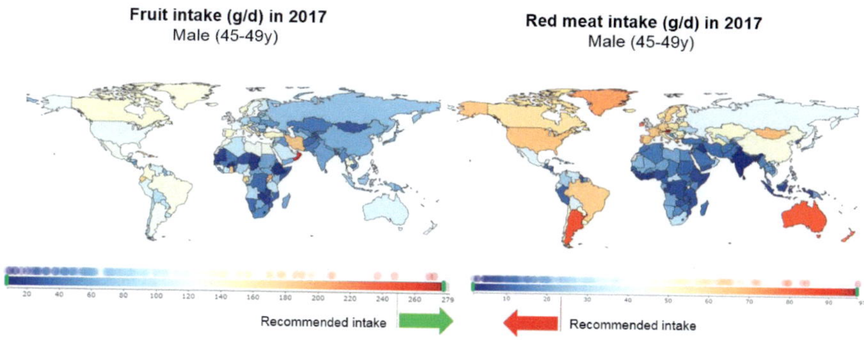

FIGURE 3-1 Population-level estimates of current intake (2017) compared with recommended intake for fruit (left) and red meat (right).
NOTE: Measurements of fruit and red meat intake are both in grams/day (g/d) and both for males aged 45 to 49, based on Global Burden of Disease modeling.
SOURCE: Presented by Ashkan Afshin on August 1, 2018.

each dietary factor. Usual intake, as opposed to 1-day intake, corrects for daily within person variation, he explained.

Other Challenges to Analyzing Dietary Data

Afshin went on to observe that, in addition to comparing and combining dietary data from different sources, there are other challenges to measuring the human diet. He briefly mentioned a few of these, beginning with how diet should be defined. Should it be defined in terms of nutrients, food, or dietary patterns? Should absolute intake or diet composition be measured? According to Afshin, different approaches and measures have different advantages and disadvantages and different implications for estimating health effects. He noted that, although GBD's focus has traditionally been on health effects, the implications differ for potential environmental impacts as well.

Afshin went on to cite as another challenge that the definition of dietary factors varies across studies. He gave the example of the definition of "whole grain," which varies widely across studies, encompassing different categories of food items (e.g., breakfast cereals, brown rice, brown rice flour, buckwheat, nonwhite bread, and oats in one study, versus added bran, added wheat germ, brown rice, brown rice flour, buckwheat, bulgur, oats, popcorn, and psyllium in another). In Afshin's opinion, whole grain is perhaps one of the most challenging food groups to define. In addition, fruit, which may seem straightforward, is in fact a highly heterogeneous food group, with different fruits having different nutrient profiles, and therefore different health and environmental impacts. Moreover, Afshin observed, people have very strong opinions about what should be considered a fruit. For example, he pointed out, some people think cucumbers, tomatoes, and eggplant are fruits, while others do not. With nuts too, he continued, some people argue for a botanical definition, yet peanuts, which are a legume, not a tree nut, are lumped together with tree nuts in the nut food group because they have identical nutrient profiles. He explained that GBD's approach to handling this challenge is to extract data at the food item level wherever such data exist and then use coding to regroup food items as necessary, depending on how the data will be used.

Afshin identified serving size as yet another challenge, particularly for food questionnaire data. He noted that a common question on food questionnaires is the number of servings an individual consumes, adding that while it might be straightforward to convert an apple serving to grams using the U.S. Department of Agriculture's (USDA's) Food Composition Database (in which one apple is 182 grams), converting a serving size of broccoli into grams depends on whether the broccoli is cooked or uncooked and on how it is consumed. Thus, he cautioned, many assumptions must be made, and for some food items, such as a pat of butter, serving size must be determined arbitrarily. He cited as another serving size challenge that defined serving size varies across studies, even in the same country. For example, a serving of salmon may be defined as 3 to 4 ounces in one study but as one can or half of a fillet in others.

Final Remarks

To summarize, Afshin highlighted five key lessons learned by GBD. First, dietary data are far from being optimal. Second, despite these limitations, multiple lines of evidence show that diet is an important risk factor for the health of people and the planet. Third, echoing one of Fanzo's key messages, Afshin said, "We cannot wait for perfect data in order to make decisions. Decisions have to be made now." Fourth, as part of GBD, methods have been developed for making the best use of current dietary data to characterize the human diet and to inform decision making. Finally, Afshin asserted that new data sources and new data processing methods should be harnessed as they become available to improve and update existing dietary estimates, something GBD does through its annual updating.

DIETARY PATTERNS LINK HUMAN HEALTH AND THE ENVIRONMENT

David Tilman, University of Minnesota, Saint Paul, began by reporting that, based on the World Health Organization's (WHO's) analyses of disease burden, it is now known that the dietary transition currently under way around the world is highly associated with declining health, especially in relation to noncommunicable diseases. Of the top 12 risks to health, he elaborated, 7 are diet-related worldwide (WHO, 2009), and 8 are in the United States (Holland, 2018). WHO projects that by 2030, noncommunicable diseases, such as diabetes, heart disease, and stroke, will account for the globally dominant disease burden (Aleksandrowicz et al., 2016).

Modern food systems are also a major cause of harm to the environment, Tilman observed, with an estimated 30 percent of global greenhouse gas (GHG) emissions coming from agricultural food production, including both crops and livestock (Aleksandrowicz et al., 2016). He called attention to two additional environmental impacts of agriculture. First, he noted that agriculture is a major cause of pollution in lakes, rivers, groundwater, and oceans (i.e., eutrophication). He pointed to the dead zone in the Gulf of Mexico as just one example. Every river in the world that drains a substantial agricultural area also has a dead zone, he added, signaling pollution of regional groundwater and harm to the quality of drinking water (Diaz and Rosenberg, 2008). He mentioned that people who live downwind of fertilized agricultural fields suffer health harms as well from exposure to fine particulate matter ($PM_{2.5}$ particles) (World Bank and IHME, 2016). The second environmental impact of agriculture beyond GHG emissions, according to Tilman, is that it is responsible for land loss that represents the major threat of extinction for species on Earth. Many ecologists would assert, he stated, that eutrophication and extinction are co-equal partners with climate change as threats to the long-term sustainability of the support systems on which humanity depends.

Tilman went on to discuss each of these three environmental impacts—GHG emissions, eutrophication, and land loss—in greater detail, while also emphasizing their links, via diet, with human health.

Food and Greenhouse Gas Emissions

Turning first to GHG emissions, Tilman cited evidence indicating clear differences in contributions to GHG emissions among different foods. He noted that plant-based products, for example, are responsible for relatively low GHG emissions (see Figure 3-2). He added that although GHG emissions attributable to various foods are plotted per kilocalorie in Figure 3-2, the same observations apply per USDA serving size and, for foods that contain protein, per gram of protein (Tilman and Clark, 2014). Thus, not only are diets with reduced amounts of red meat associated with reductions in diabetes, cancers, heart disease, and all-cause mortality compared with a typical westernized diet (see Figure 3-3), but they also are associated with lower amounts of GHG emissions (see Figure 3-4). "Adoption of these diets

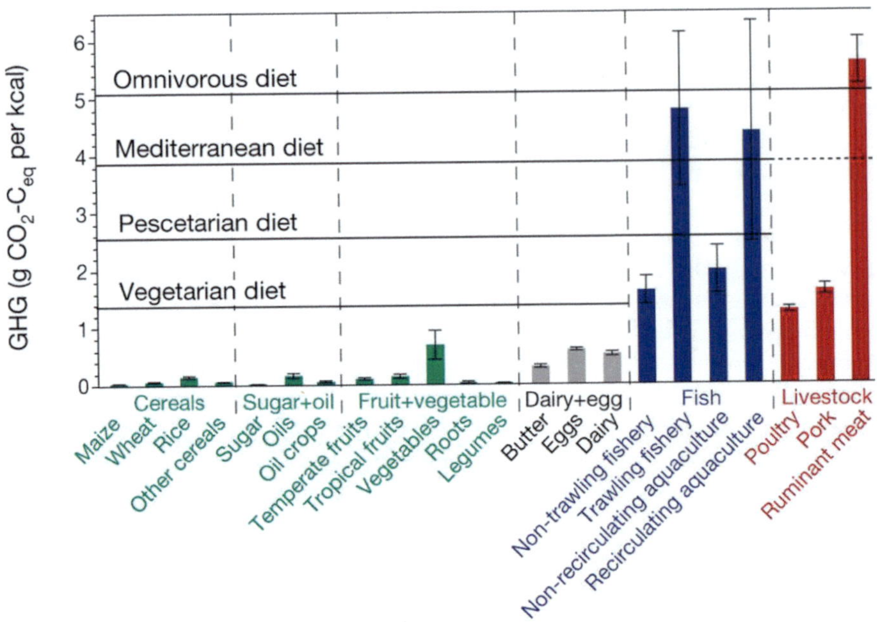

FIGURE 3-2 Greenhouse gas (GHG) impacts for a range of foods.
NOTE: GHG is measured in grams of carbon dioxide (CO_2)-equivalent per kilocalorie (kcal).
SOURCES: Presented by David Tilman on August 1, 2018, modified from Tilman and Clark, 2014.

around the world could have huge implications," Tilman argued (Tilman and Clark, 2014).

Tilman went on to state that by 2050, if current dietary trends toward consumption of more meat, more calories, and more empty calories continue, equivalent global carbon dioxide (CO_2) emissions from crop production are expected to increase by about 2 gigatons (Gt) per year when measured in terms of the mass of carbon (C) (Tilman and Clark, 2014). He added that this figure is equivalent to increased annual global emissions of about 7.5 Gt of CO_2, a little more than what is currently emitted by all transportation worldwide. "But if people adopted Mediterranean, pescetarian, or vegetarian diets," he argued, "we could have ... lower emissions in 2050 from agricultural food production than we have right now from it. Diet can be a big lever." He pointed out, however, that while diet is a big lever, it is not the only lever for addressing sustainable diets, and he then turned to how crops are grown and the precision and efficiency of fertilizer and irrigation.

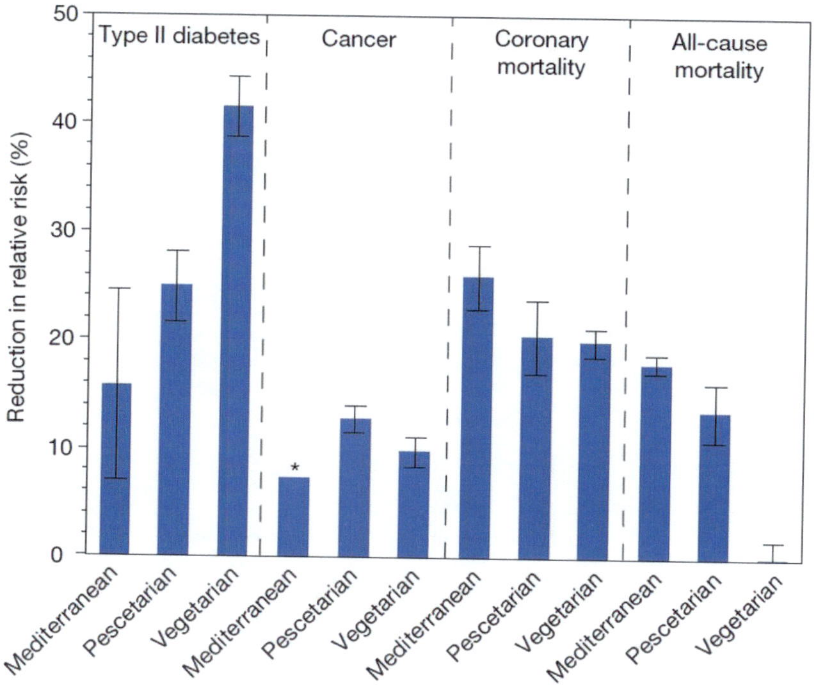

FIGURE 3-3 Diet-dependent percentage reductions in relative risk of various health outcomes for alternative diets (Mediterranean, pescetarian, and vegetarian) compared with the conventional omnivorous diet.
SOURCES: Presented by David Tilman on August 1, 2018, modified from Tilman and Clark, 2014.

Food and Eutrophication

According to Tilman, the eutrophication impacts of agriculture, especially nitrogen pollution of surface water, lakes, rivers, and streams, could increase by 70 percent or more over the next 50 years (Tilman et al., 2001). He noted that other researchers have put forth estimates of 100 percent or more. He remarked that people often think of maize as having a very high eutrophication effect, with leftover nutrients from the corn being grown in the United States draining down the Mississippi River and creating the dead zone in the Gulf of Mexico. Yet, he asserted, "this is nothing compared to beef." He explained that the eutrophication potential of ruminant meat (per calorie) is much greater than that of maize because it takes about 15 kilograms of protein from grains to make 1 kilogram of edible beef protein. Thus, similar to the pattern depicted in Figure 3-2 with respect to GHGs, plant-based diets also have lower per capita eutrophication effects (Tilman and Clark, 2014).

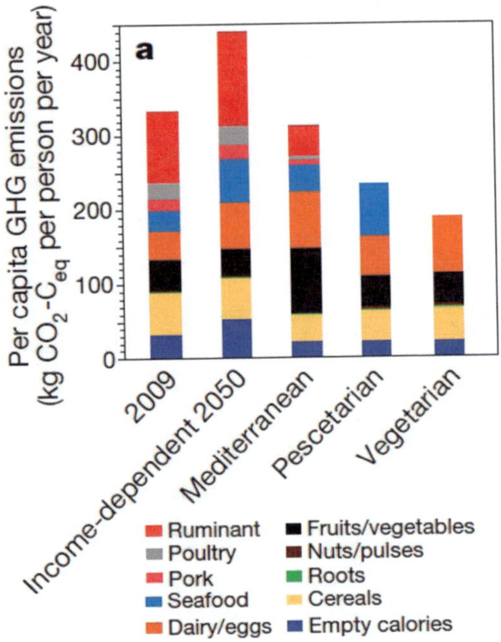

FIGURE 3-4 Per capita greenhouse gas (GHG) emissions for five diets (2009 global average, 2050 global income-dependent, Mediterranean, pescetarian, and vegetarian).
NOTE: GHG is measured in grams of carbon dioxide (CO_2)-equivalent per kilocalorie per person per year.
SOURCES: Presented by David Tilman on August 1, 2018, modified from Tilman and Clark, 2014.

Another way to visualize the relationship between diet and eutrophication, Tilman continued, is to plot eutrophication impact against the relative risk of health impact. Again, he remarked, for unprocessed foods there is a clear relationship between the two: a linear change in food group–associated health impacts is associated with an exponential change in food group–associated eutrophication impact. For example, according to the data he shared, not only do whole grains pose the lowest relative mortality risk, but they also have among the smallest eutrophication impacts (Clark, 2018), and a dietary change that would reduce overall relative mortality risk from 1.5 to 0.85 would, on average, cause a 100-fold reduction in eutrophication impact. Tilman interpreted these results to mean that the dietary changes with "personally huge health impacts have even greater environmental impacts."

But again, Tilman observed, diet is not the only lever. He mentioned the large body of research demonstrating how agricultural yields can be retained with the use of roughly 20 percent less fertilizer if the fertilizer is applied more precisely—in other words, the right amount at the right time for a crop. To illustrate, he noted that crop yields (tons of protein per hectacre per year) in France, Germany, Italy, and Mexico increased from 1950 through 2009 even though nitrogen use (i.e., fertilization per hectacre) declined because of both new farm policies and higher fertilizer costs (FAO, 2009).

Food and Extinction of Species

An analysis by the International Union for Conservation of Nature (IUCN) of all mammal and bird species worldwide, Tilman continued, found that the single greatest factor threatening species with extinction is land clearing, particularly land cleared for agriculture. The next-greatest threat, he reported, is logging, most of which is occurring in tropical countries; after being logged, such lands often become pastures or croplands. He identified direct hunting for food as the third-greatest threat to species extinction worldwide (Tilman et al., 2017).

Tilman went on to observe that most of the Earth's remaining large mammals (i.e., larger than 10 kilograms, a bit larger than a small dog) inhabit the southern part of Asia, tropical Asia, and tropical Africa (see Figure 3-5). He added that the percentage of large mammals in sub-Saharan Africa that is threatened with extinction is relatively low compared with the percentage in southern Asia—as great as 60 to 85 percent (Tilman et al., 2017).

"But we have a world that is growing," Tilman continued. According to the United Nations, there will be 1.7 billion more people living in sub-Saharan Africa in the next 50 years. This is also an area with rapidly growing economies, he observed, with people purchasing and consuming more food as their incomes rise. In fact, this trend occurs globally, with calories per day increasing as income rises (Tilman et al., 2017) (see Figure 3-6). Demand for meat shows a similar pattern. Tilman again mentioned that it takes about 15 kilograms of grain protein to produce 1 kilogram of edible beef and about 4 kilograms of grain protein to produce 1 kilogram of edible chicken. Thus, he noted, about 8,000 calories of crops must be grown per person per day to provide the approximately 3,500 calories of food that are brought into the home daily (per capita) and the 2,500 to 3,000 calories actually consumed (again, per capita) in a wealthy nation. According to Tilman, the net effect of the growing global population, taken together with the income-dependent dietary shift toward more calories—more meat calories in particular—and more crops to support production of those calories, will be about a 70 to 100 percent increase in global food production over the next 50 years. Based on the impact of this increased

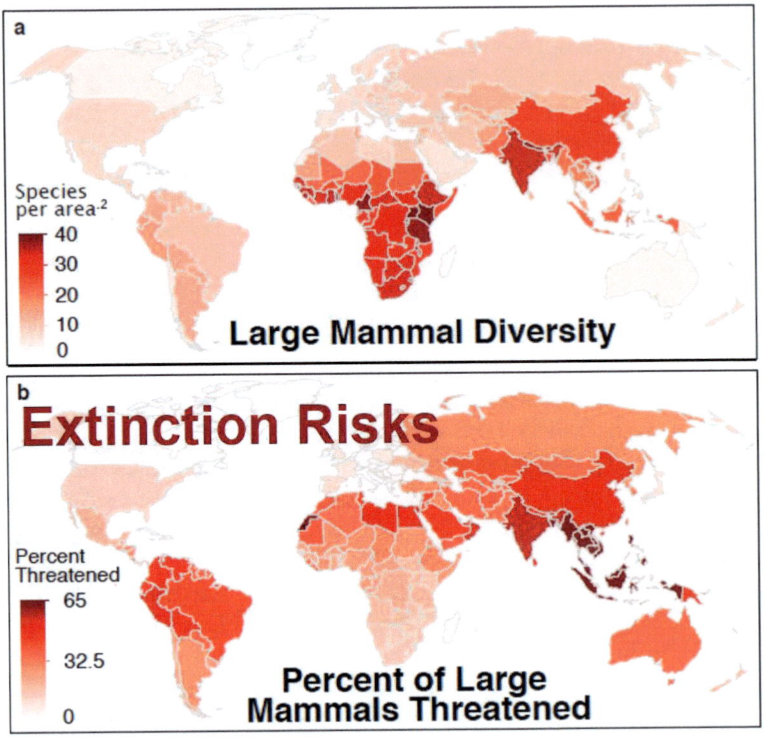

FIGURE 3-5 Large-mammal (>10 kg) diversity worldwide (top map) and percentage of large mammals threated with extinction (bottom map).
SOURCES: Presented by David Tilman on August 1, 2018, modified from Tilman et al., 2017.

agricultural production on land clearing predicted by Tilman and colleagues (2017), the extinction risk for large mammals will double in Asia, dramatically increase in sub-Saharan Africa, and increase markedly in South America during this time period.

"The good news is that diet can help prevent some of this," Tilman stated. Conversion of tropical ecosystems into cropland could be prevented, he argued, if people adopted more plant-based diets relative to today's trends. For example, he suggested, about 600 million hectares of land could be saved if everyone converted to a vegetarian diet, and slightly less for a pescetarian diet (about 550 million hectares) or Mediterranean diet (about 450 million hectares) (Tilman and Clark, 2014). He pointed out that 600 million hectares is about two-thirds of the area of the United States and asserted that preventing that much land from being destroyed would have a major biodiversity benefit.

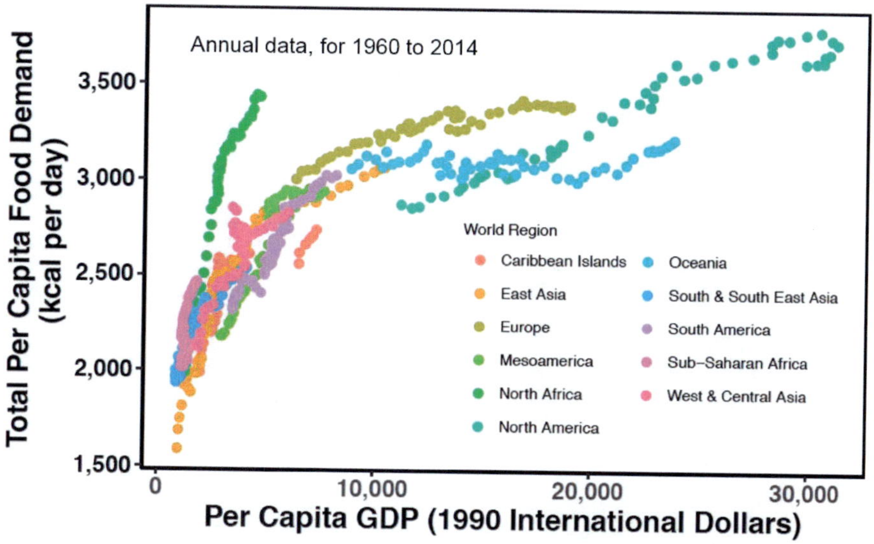

FIGURE 3-6 Per capita calories brought into homes daily as a function of income (per capita gross domestic product [GDP]) for different regions of the world, 1960–2014.
SOURCES: Presented by David Tilman on August 1, 2018, modified from Tilman et al., 2011.

In addition to diet, Tilman emphasized the powerful role of trade in preserving land that serves as a natural ecosystem. In fact, he suggested, if done to minimize future land clearing, exports of crops from nations with higher yields to those with lower yields might prevent about as much land clearing as could be forestalled by dietary shifts (Tilman et al., 2017) (see Figure 3-7).

Final Remarks

To summarize, Tilman described recent, unpublished work revealing a fairly tight log-linear relationship between diet-related health effects (mortality, heart disease, diabetes, and stroke) and diet-related environmental impacts across four different areas (GHG emissions, eutrophication, use of irrigation water, and land clearing). He interpreted these results to mean that even a relatively small shift toward healthier, more plant-based diets would have both health benefits and even larger environmental benefits. He noted, however, that there are some outliers, one being sugar-sweetened beverages, observing that foods with added sugars have relatively low environmental impacts but negative health impacts. On average, however, with some exceptions, "healthier foods offer greater environmental benefits," he concluded.

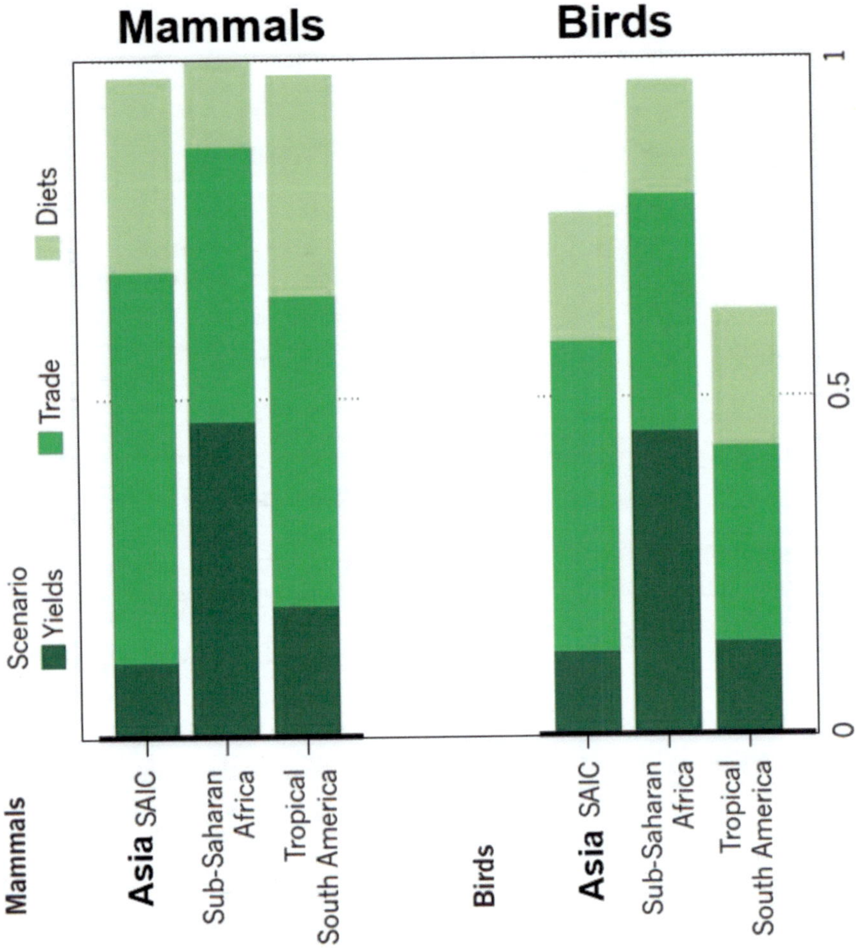

FIGURE 3-7 Predicted reductions in extinction risk for birds and mammals in different regions of the world as a result of dietary shifts that prevent land clearing, increased trade of crops from nations with higher yields to nations with lower yields, and increased yields.
NOTES: SAIC = Southeast Asia, India, and China. Dietary shifts that prevent land clearing are depicted by upper lightly shaded bars; increased trade of crops from nations with higher yields to nations with lower yields are depicted by middle bars; and dietary shifts that increase yields are depicted by lower darkly shaded bars.
SOURCES: Presented by David Tilman on August 1, 2018, modified from Tilman et al., 2017.

WHAT MAKES FOR FOOD SYSTEMS THAT ARE SUSTAINABLE AND RESILIENT?

Mark Rosegrant, International Food Policy Research Institute (IFPRI), Washington, DC, offered a definition of sustainability similar to but slightly different from the 2012 FAO definition cited earlier by Drewnowski and others (see Chapter 2), but still a UN definition: "A sustainable food system is a food system that delivers food and nutrition security for all in such a way that the economic, social, and environmental bases to generate food security and nutrition for future generations are not compromised" (HLPE, 2017). In addition, he defined a resilient food system as "a system that is able to persist, adapt, and transform under conditions of uncertainty" (Folke et al., 2010). Starting with these definitions, he stated that the objective of his presentation would be to explore what policies, investments, and behavioral changes contribute to improving income, food security, and nutrition while reducing GHG emissions, the use of water and land, and the conversion of forests.

Challenges to Sustainable, Resilient Food Systems

Elaborating on points made by several other speakers, Rosegrant identified several challenges to achieving a sustainable diet, as detailed below.

Increasing Prevalence of Overweight and Obesity

Rosegrant observed that the world has been experiencing a slow decline in malnourishment, down from about 1 billion malnourished people worldwide in the 1990s to 800 million currently. Moreover, the number of stunted children worldwide has decreased as well over that same time period, although mostly in Asia, with the number in Africa increasing. But simultaneously, Rosegrant pointed out, there has been a rapid increase in the number of overweight and obese children worldwide, including in Africa and Asia (de Onis et al., 2010, 2012).

Pervasive Micronutrient Deficiencies

In addition to the rapid rise in obesity, Rosegrant cited pervasive micronutrient deficiencies, including extreme cumulative deficiencies in India and other parts of Asia, and medium to high cumulative deficiencies in much of the rest of Asia as well (FAO, 2013a). Citing a specific example, he reported that the economic cost of micronutrient deficiencies in India has been estimated at US$17.3 billion (2004 dollars), or 2.5 percent of India's gross domestic product (GDP) (Stein and Qaim, 2007). He added that, according to FAO data, there is a high prevalence of specific micronutrient deficiencies worldwide as well (e.g., anemia, vitamin A deficiency, iodine deficiency) (FAO, 2013a).

Population Growth and Urbanization

Rosegrant observed that the United Nations has projected rapid population growth in sub-Saharan Africa, South Asia, and East Asia in particular (see Figure 3-8). Those same areas are also the most challenged nutritionally with respect to food security, he pointed out. Also as shown in Figure 3-8, the world is becoming more urbanized (UNDESA, 2014), with the implications discussed below.

Evolving Food Demand: Increasing Consumption of Sugar, Fats, Oils, and Meat

Rosegrant described the several ways in which food demand is evolving as a result of urbanization and rapid income growth. While diets are changing in some positive ways—for example, he noted that the consumption of fruits and vegetables is increasing in much of the world—consumption

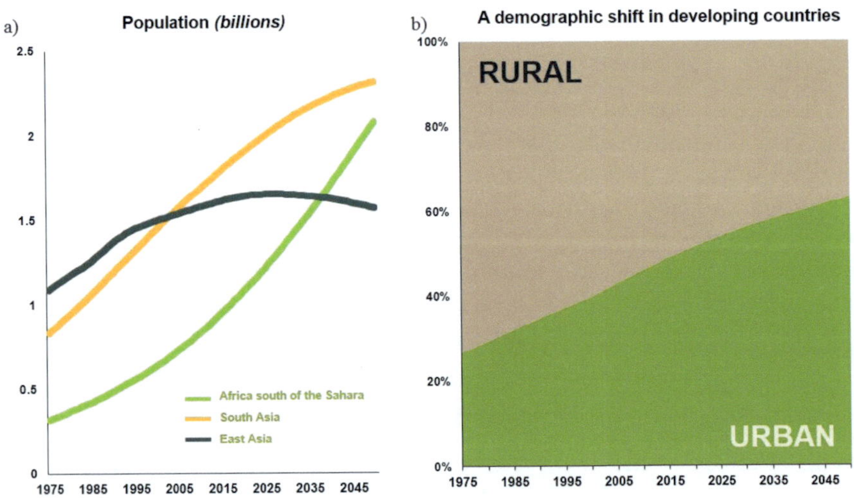

FIGURE 3-8 (a) Projected population growth in Africa and South Asia through 2050. (b) Projected demographic shift in developing countries to a more urbanized world, through 2050.
NOTE: Population growth is depicted in billions.
SOURCES: Presented by Mark Rosegrant on August 1, 2018, based on information from UN World Urbanization Prospects, 2014 revision.

of sugar, fats, and oils is also increasing, and people are eating more convenience and fast foods. In addition, he observed, meat consumption continues to grow rapidly, leading to a rapidly growing demand for grains for feed. According to Rosegrant, half of the growth in grain demand through 2050 is likely to be for the direct feeding of livestock. "That, in turn," he said, "puts intense pressure, of course, on land and water" (IFPRI, 2011).

Water Stress and Crop Yield

In 2011, work by Rosegrant and his IFPRI colleagues, in collaboration with the Veolia Water Company, found that 36 percent of the global population lived in a water-scarce area and that 39 percent of global grain production and 22 percent of global GDP were located in areas with significant water stress. By 2050, Rosegrant reported, these numbers are expected to be much higher, with half the population (52 percent), half of grain production (49 percent), and nearly half of global GDP (45 percent) occupying water-stressed regions (FAO, 2011; IFPRI, 2011).

Regarding crop yields, Rosegrant continued, yields of maize are projected to be 30 percent lower in 2050 than today because of climate change, compared with no climate change (Nelson et al., 2009). Thus, he stated, much of the world, including the United States, will experience heavy losses in yield. He pointed out that U.S. yield and exports play an important role in global food security.

International Food Policy Research Institute's (IFPRI's) International Model for Policy Analysis of Agricultural Commodities and Trade (IMPACT): Comparing Future Impacts of Different Climate Change, Agricultural Investment, and Meat Demand Scenarios

Rosegrant described how, given the above challenges, IFPRI's IMPACT modeling system has been used to examine and compare several different future climate change, agricultural investment, and meat demand scenarios. Without going into great detail, he described IMPACT as a global, multimarket model with a high level of disaggregation, encompassing 159 countries, 154 water basins, and 60 commodities (Robinson et al., 2015). The model links climate, water, and crop models, capturing macroeconomic and sectoral trends as well, including GDP and income growth, although modelers can specify alternative assumptions. In the version discussed by Rosegrant, IMPACT is also linked to a general equilibrium model that captures the effects of economic changes (e.g., changes in labor, employment, and GDP) on the agricultural sector (Robinson et al., 2015).

As outputs, Rosegrant continued, IMPACT generates estimates of yields, commodity prices, trade, employment, household income annually, and other impacts. Through the use of postsolution models, indicators of hunger, nutrition, and health can also be estimated. Rosegrant shared results, detailed below, for two postsolution indicators: number of hungry people (using FAO methodology to estimate the number of people below a specific calorie consumption threshold in any given country) and number of stunted children (based on econometric results estimated by Lisa Smith and Lawrence Haddad[1]). Rosegrant explained that all of these results were based on the most severe representative concentration pathway (RCP) climate change scenario (the Intergovernmental Panel on Climate Change's [IPCC's] RCP of 8.5), plus a medium level of GDP growth.

Scenarios for More Sustainable and Resilient Food Systems: Investing in Agricultural Efficiency

First, Rosegrant described results from modeling three different types of additional investments in the agricultural sector to improve productivity and efficiency: (1) research and development investments to increase productivity, including investments by CGIAR, a global partnership and the main international agricultural research system, as well as investments by the National Agricultural Research System (NARS); (2) various water investments, including the expansion of irrigation systems, the enhancement of water use efficiency, and enhanced soil management (e.g., system-level efficiency, no-till farming, integrated soil fertility management, and rainwater harvesting); and (3) investments in rural infrastructure to benefit agricultural production and value chains (e.g., investments in the transportation and energy sectors).

Rosegrant and colleagues modeled the impacts of each of the sets of investments separately and then the impacts of all together (the "comprehensive investment portfolio"). According to Rosegrant, the comprehensive investment portfolio totaled about \$25.5 billion per year above baseline (current annual expenditures are about \$38 billion). The researchers ran the models from 2015 through 2050. They examined three different types of outcomes in 2050, all computed relative to baseline: (1) income (GDP per capita); (2) outcomes related to food supply, hunger, and nutrition (agricultural supply, hunger, stunted children); and (3) environment (water use, GHG emissions, forest cover).

In the interest of time, Rosegrant described only the results of the comprehensive investment scenario. The researchers were essentially asking, in that scenario, with all of these various additional annual investments totaling \$25.5 billion per year above baseline beginning in 2015, how outcomes

[1]For more information, see https://www.sciencedirect.com/science/article/pii/S0305750X14003726 (accessed January 7, 2019).

in 2050 would be different compared with the baseline investment level. The model projected a nearly 6 percent increase in per capita income in 2050 due to higher investment compared with the baseline scenario, Rosegrant reported. In addition, as expected, it projected a substantial increase in agricultural supply (11.5 percent), a 24 percent reduction in hunger, and a 9 percent reduction in the number of stunted children in 2050 compared with the baseline investment. In other words, he clarified, there would be 120 million fewer hungry people and 10 million fewer stunted children in 2050 as a result of these additional agricultural investments. With respect to environmental outcomes, he added, these investments would generate substantial reductions in water use—about 11 percent. In addition, because both crop and livestock productivity would be enhanced, land use would also be reduced, with about 88 million hectares saved. The more efficient production of animals with respect to methane gases would generate a reduction of about 25 percent in GHG emissions, or about 3 Gt, by 2050.

Scenarios for More Sustainable and Resilient Food Systems: Reduced Meat Demand

The IMPACT modeling system was also used to predict future outcomes under different reduced meat demand scenarios, Rosegrant continued. One of these scenarios was a high-income scenario involving a 50 percent reduction in per capita meat demand in all high-income countries relative to baseline (i.e., no meat reduction). Another scenario was a 50 percent reduction in both high-income countries and the two of the largest middle-income countries, Brazil and China. One of the important findings from this modeling exercise, Rosegrant pointed out, was that when meat consumption was reduced in both the high-income countries and Brazil and China, it increased dramatically in sub-Saharan Africa—more than 30 percent over its current very low levels (see Figure 3-9). Meat consumption increased dramatically among developing countries overall (minus Brazil and China) as well, by a little less than 30 percent. Rosegrant explained that these increases were projected to occur elsewhere in the world because of the lower prices due to the reduced consumption of meat. The other finding of note, he said, was that the impacts of a reduction in Brazil and China were even greater than the impacts of a reduction in high-income countries because of those two countries' large populations, coupled with their high levels of meat consumption.

According to Rosegrant, the model also revealed reduced demand for feed grain and a modest reduction in the risk of hunger. The latter finding, he explained, was the result of not only lower-priced meats but also lower-priced grains, particularly maize, but also wheat and rice, inducing people to increase their consumption. When both high-income countries

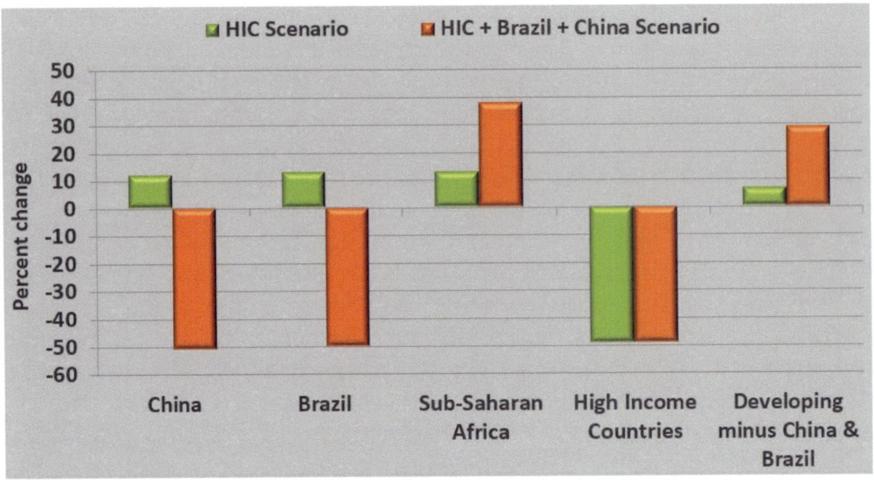

FIGURE 3-9 Percentage change in meat consumption projected from the International Food Policy Research Institute's (IFPRI's) International Model for Policy Analysis of Agricultural Commodities and Trade (IMPACT) modeling of a forced 50 percent reduction in meat consumption from 2015 to 2050 in high-income countries (HICs) or both in HICs and in Brazil and China.
NOTES: HICs are depicted by green bars. HICs and Brazil and China are depicted by orange bars.
SOURCE: Presented by Mark Rosegrant on August 1, 2018.

and Brazil and China reduced meat consumption, the risk of hunger in sub-Saharan Africa and developing countries overall was reduced by 9 and 6 percent, respectively. In terms of absolute numbers, Rosegrant elaborated, this reduction would bring 60 million people out of hunger in developing countries, 40 million of them in sub-Saharan Africa. Again, he said, these results point to "important distributional impacts from that drop in meat consumption."

In both of the scenarios with reduced meat consumption, Rosegrant added, significant land would also be conserved, including both cropland and pasture. Under the scenario involving high-income countries plus Brazil and China, a total of 180 million hectares of land worldwide would be saved. Land in developing countries, minus Brazil and China, would account for a little less than half of that total.

For purposes of comparison, Rosegrant mentioned results from a different modeling study, in which non-CO_2 GHG emissions were examined under three different meat demand scenarios (constant, more, and less) (Popp et al., 2010). By 2060, GHG emissions were projected to increase by about 40 percent in the constant meat demand scenario, compared with about a 60 percent increase at baseline (i.e., no meat reduction) in Rosegrant and colleagues' IMPACT modeling. In the more meat demand scenario, GHG emissions doubled. In the less meat demand scenario, GHG emissions decreased by about 60 percent, which Rosegrant noted was similar to what he and his colleagues had observed with the IMPACT model. So again, Rosegrant observed, reduced meat consumption was projected to have very large impacts on GHG emissions.

Final Remarks

In conclusion, Rosegrant summarized three main points. First, increased investment in agricultural research and development, rural infrastructure, and irrigation and water use efficiency would generate substantial increases or improvements in food supply, income, food security, and nutrition. Rosegrant emphasized, however, that the income necessary for improving food security and nutrition can be generated only with increased food production in developing countries. "You are not going to get that kind of income improvement by importing food," he said, adding that more efficient agriculture also results in reduced water use, GHG emissions, and forest loss. Second, dietary change policies could also be powerful, and arguably more so, in reducing GHG emissions, hunger, and agricultural land use. And third, achieving more resilient, sustainable food systems will require a balanced approach and recognition of the need for sustainable productivity growth, improved value chains, and significant dietary changes.

DISCUSSION

Following Rosegrant's presentation, he, Afshin, and Tilman participated in an open discussion with the audience, summarized here.

Modeling for Resilience

In reference to Rosegrant's consideration of not just sustainable but also resilient food systems, Nicole Tichenor Blackstone asked about ways in which modeling can capture the different dimensions of resiliency in a robust way across different contexts. Rosegrant clarified that IMPACT captures resilience in the sense, for example, that expanding irrigation while also increasing the efficiency of water use provides additional resilience for farmers, who then need not rely on rainwater. However, he agreed that much more could be done with IMPACT to explore resilience. In addition, he mentioned work with which he has been involved in collaboration with The World Bank on the short-term impacts of El Niño Southern Oscillation (ENSO) events (El Niño and La Niña) and the types of policy responses available.

Tilman agreed that irrigation is "incredibly important" for ensuring resiliency, particularly in areas of periodic drought. In addition, he mentioned work in his lab on patterns of crop production worldwide suggesting that greater local crop diversity on farms appears to be associated with more resiliency. Thus, he suggested that diversity may be another component of resiliency in agriculture.

Modeling for Meat Versus Protein Versus Fish

Maha Tahiri asked Rosegrant whether he had modeled for protein overall, not just for meat, and projected outcomes by 2050 if everyone worldwide simply met the recommended level of protein intake. Rosegrant replied that he and his colleagues have not yet done this modeling, although they now have the capability to do so not just for protein but for about 15 other nutrients as well. The list of nutrients on which they will focus is still being finalized, he noted, based on input from a team of nutritionists. He expects that input to be available quite soon.

Tahiri then asked Tilman to explain the variation in environmental impacts of fish (shown earlier in Figure 3-2). Tilman clarified that wild-caught fish caught on "long lines" with hooks have very low GHG impact ("non-trawling fishery" in Figure 3-2). In contrast, trawling, which basically involves dragging nets deep in the ocean, often along the ocean floor, requires boats to use much more diesel fuel ("trawling fishery" in Figure 3-2). Tilman explained that the amount of GHGs emitted by trawling fisheries is about halfway between what is emitted by chicken and beef production. Fish grown in ponds or nets suspended in the ocean are associated with higher GHG emissions, he noted, similar to those of chicken, but if aquaculture uses pumps to recirculate and filter the water, emissions can be similar to those of trawling fisheries because of the energy required of the pumps ("recirculating aquaculture" in Figure 3-2). Thus, he summarized, fish can be either low- or high-impact, depending on how they are caught or produced (Tilman and Clark, 2014).

Food Safety and Sustainability

Jessica Campbell of General Mills asked whether and where food safety is being considered in discussions of sustainable diets. In the GBD study, Afshin replied, the assumption is that food safety causes an immediate, not a long-term, effect, and thus it has not been incorporated into his team's analyses of overall health effects. He said he recognizes, however, that there are different opinions as to whether such factors as trans-fat intake are food safety issues. If the definition of food safety is expanded to include such factors, he explained, then yes, some aspects of food safety are included in the work he and his team do.

Errors of the Estimates

Johanna Dwyer, National Institutes of Health, asked about the size of the errors of the various estimates discussed by the speakers and how those errors are estimated.

Afshin replied that in GBD, the researchers work with about 20 risk factors that are all related to some form of malnutrition—either undernutrition (stunting, wasting, micronutrient deficiencies), diet quality or composition, or excess calorie intake (overweight, obesity). One of the current challenges, he observed, is how to account for overlap when combining all of these risk factors and all of their effects to derive a single diet-related burden of disease. To this end, he explained, he and his team developed metrics for estimating direct versus mediated effects—an effect could be partly a direct effect of diet but also partly mediated, for example, through obesity. He noted that a paper describing this work is forthcoming. With respect to the risk factor estimates themselves, he continued, estimates for micronutrient deficiencies, for instance, have been very unstable because of the assumptions that must be made about daily versus usual intake. He mentioned that GBD has been working with FAO to reevaluate estimates of micronutrient deficiency. As an example, he explained that when results were corrected for daily variation in zinc intake, the prevalence of zinc deficiency dropped from about 20 to 25 percent to less than 10 percent.

With the IMPACT modeling system, Rosegrant said, IFPRI has been unable to establish formal error bands because of the number of variables. He noted, however, that his team has done some backcasting, the results of which have suggested that their regional predictions have been fairly accurate and in some places, such as China, "spot on."

Language: Use of the Term "Processed Food"

"I think it is very important as we proceed in this conversation, with lots of different people from different disciplines coming together, that words matter," Kristi Reimers, Conagra Brands, commented. She mentioned the pervasiveness of using "processed food" as a surrogate for high-energy-dense, low-nutrient-dense foods. She said she understood that it is difficult to say "high-energy-dense, low-nutrient-dense," but suggested that a different surrogate be used, as not all processed foods can be thus characterized. As an example, she pointed to tomatoes that are processed during tomato season, so they are a processed food, but a very high-nutrient-dense food. She suggested that a different surrogate could help with more effective communication.

Red Meat: How to Move Forward Other Than Saying "Eat Less"

"It is very hard to create a positive story for red meat when we talk about sustainability," Reimers continued. The increase in demand for red meat continues, she observed, still outselling vegan or vegetarian options "hands down." She stressed that this demand cannot be ignored, and asked whether there are other solutions besides telling people to "eat less."

In Tilman's opinion, this is a fundamental question. He mentioned human evolutionary history, with meat being an important part of humans' diets when they lived as hunter–gatherers. He believes that much of the current conversation around sustainable diets stems from a fundamental conflict between the taste preference humans have for items that were limited in their evolutionary past, such as salt, sugar, fats, and proteins, and the foods that are actually healthy for them and the environment. These taste preferences, he asserted, can lead people to like manufactured foods that have unhealthy levels of salt, sugar, and fat and to eat more red meat than is healthy. He argued for putting more effort into developing foods that are nutritionally dense and lower in calories but also very high in what humans perceive as good taste. He pointed out that vegetarian and vegan foods can be delicious and suggested that some entrepreneurs or companies invest in making what he described as "incredibly delicious varieties of such foods." He predicted that there could be a much greater market for these tasty and healthy foods.

Rosegrant mentioned the surprisingly rapid development of "clean meat," which is laboratory-developed meat cloned from cells. In his opinion, its taste is almost as satisfying as that of regular meat. However, he predicted that it would take perhaps another 10 to 15 years before clean meat can compete with regular meat.

Instead of focusing on preferences, Rosegrant suggested, another strategy is to use punitive taxes, either carbon taxes, which would be far higher for meat than for other, healthier foods, or direct meat taxes. He acknowledged, however, that such taxes would be a "tough sell" in a country such as the United States, and that in most of Africa and much of Asia, where people are eating only 1 to 2 kilograms of meat per capita daily, even substantial increases in meat consumption could be beneficial.

Wilde added that in the United States, the meat industry has almost a veto power over certain proposals or strategies that are particularly harmful to meat industry–related livelihoods. At first glance and compared with baseline, he observed, some of Rosegrant's results might look fairly frightening to someone in the meat industry. He wondered, however, whether the results were really as "bad" as they looked. For Wilde, one of the more interesting modeling results described by Rosegrant during his presentation was the increased consumption in other parts of the world when prices fell in currently high meat-consuming countries. He suggested that this increased consumption elsewhere could be developed into an acceptable storyline for those in the meat industry who want to be "good sports" about sustainable diets but have some line below which they are not willing to go.

Rosegrant explained how the models that he described supported Wilde's argument. At baseline there was about a 60 percent increase in meat consumption between 2015 and 2050. However, when meat consumption in high-income countries plus Brazil and China was reduced by 50 percent, there would still be a 10 percent increase globally by 2050 because when that much demand is removed from the global meat system, prices fall, making meat more affordable for more people (Tilman and Clark, 2014).

Data, Analysis, and Policy

Rose asked the panelists what new developments they foresee in the next few years that will affect their impressions of sustainable diets or what new developments they would like to see.

Tilman echoed what Fanzo had said earlier (see Chapter 2): that enough is known "in broad outline"; the results are large enough and the error limits small enough. "What we really need to do," he said, "is find ways to change society so that we adopt the ideas that we are talking about"—that is, make diets healthier and reduce their environmental impacts. Although he acknowledged that more data could be gathered and more intricate analyses conducted, he believes data and analyses are not the limitations. "I think we are really policy and adoption limited," he said. "That is where we need the greatest creativity."

Rosegrant replied that models could "get fancier," and in fact, he and his group are using machine learning to develop more integrated, larger models. But more important than developing new models, in his opinion, is developing more precise analytic techniques that can provide highly spatially disaggregated and real-time data that help farmers become more efficient through the use of less fertilizer and water. It is in that realm, he argued, rather than in modeling per se, that new developments could have beneficial effects.

Afshin echoed Rosegrant's call for more precise data collection methods, but in the realm of sensor-based, individual-level data. "We really do not know what people eat," he said. "We are making educated guesses."

4

Sustainability and Healthy Dietary Changes Through Policy and Program Action

In Session 3, moderated by David Klurfeld, U.S. Department of Agriculture (USDA), Beltsville, Maryland, speakers continued to explore program and policy actions that could support sustainable diets, based not just on modeling but on a variety of other types of studies as well. This chapter summarizes the presentations and discussion that took place, with highlights of the presentations provided in Box 4-1.

THE HEALTH AND ENVIRONMENTAL ASPECTS OF DIETARY CHANGES TOWARD SUSTAINABLE DIETS

Citing the same Food and Agriculture Organization (FAO) definition of sustainable diets referenced by other speakers (FAO, 2012b; see Box 2-2 in Chapter 2), Marco Springmann, Oxford University, United Kingdom, began by remarking that he would be addressing only two of the several dimensions of sustainable diets: human health and the environment.

Regarding the health impacts of food consumption, Springmann highlighted that, according to 2015 Global Burden of Disease (GBD) data, imbalanced diets are responsible for the greatest health burden globally and in most regions as well. (See Chapter 3 for a discussion of how GBD analyzes human dietary data.) Food insecurity remains a pertinent problem as well, he observed, with 2 billion people worldwide being overweight or obese, another 2 billion having nutritional deficiencies, and 800 million experiencing hunger due to poverty and poorly developed food systems (FAO et al., 2018). He stressed that the situation is expected to become worse if nothing

BOX 4-1
Highlights of Individual Presentations*

- Most research on sustainable diets and food systems centers around national case studies, with each study taking a different approach. These different approaches make it difficult to make sense of the totality of evidence. (Springmann)
  - Results of a combined analysis of health and environmental impacts of three sustainable diet strategies for 158 countries indicated that changing dietary patterns (balancing both nutrient composition and energy) shows the most promise. (Springmann)
  - Still, there are trade-offs. When these data were analyzed regionally, this same strategy had different effects in high- and middle-income versus low-income countries. (Springmann)
- Modeling work has shown that it is possible to have a diet that meets all nutrient requirements, is affordable, and has a reduced carbon footprint. But these models do not account for taste. People do not eat just for health reasons or for protection of the environment. (Macdiarmid)
  - Recommendations for sustainable diets will likely get "stuck" at the guideline stage if more thought is not given to understanding what drives people to eat what they eat. (Macdiarmid)
  - A range of plant-based diets can reduce the food system's environmental footprint. (Macdiarmid)
- There is no "silver bullet" for achieving sustainable diets. Rather, an entire menu of solutions needs to be on the table, from production strategies (e.g., improving crop breeding to increase yields, improving soil and water management, increasing livestock and pasture productivity) to consumption strategies (e.g., reducing food waste, shifting diets, and avoiding competition for land from biofuels). (Ranganathan)

is done to reverse the dietary transition currently under way (Alexandratos and Bruinsma, 2012; Springmann et al., 2016b). Regarding the environmental dimension of sustainable diets, Springmann noted that food production is a major driver of climate change (Vermeulen et al., 2012); land use change and loss of biodiversity (Houghton et al., 2012; Ramankutty et al., 2008); freshwater extraction (WWAP, 2012); and fertilizer runoff and dead zones (Diaz and Rosenberg, 2008; Vitousek et al., 1997).

In light of these findings, and given the number of systematic reviews of this evidence that are beginning to appear (Aleksandrowicz et al., 2016; Hallström et al., 2015; Joyce et al., 2012; Nelson et al., 2016), Springmann believes the sustainable diet literature has reached what he described as a

  - There are lessons to be learned from private-sector marketing about strategies that may be useful for shifting diets toward more sustainable and healthy food choices (e.g., minimizing disruption to consumers, selling a compelling benefit, maximizing awareness). (Ranganathan)
  - There are also strategies that can be applied in the food services sector that can help shift diets (e.g., the language used to describe vegetable dishes on menus can influence food choices). (Ranganathan)
- Historically, food chain interventions have focused on increasing yield and the well-being of the farmer. A nutrition-sensitive value chain (NSVC) adds nutritional value to every step of the chain, so the focus is not just on economic value. (Tahiri)
  - There is as yet no evidence from randomized controlled trials comparing NSVCs with traditional interventions, but there is proof of concept. (Tahiri)
  - Among other factors, success requires a clear definition of the nutrition problem and goal, as well as added value for all stakeholders. (Tahiri)
- There are multiple opportunities for integrating sustainability into each of the three essential functions of the *Dietary Guidelines for Americans* (DGA) process. (Schneeman)
  - During strategic planning, sustainability could be made an explicit part of the purpose statement, and sustainability topics relevant to the DGA could be identified for future consideration. (Schneeman)
  - In both the analysis and synthesis/interpretation phases, experts with the relevant sustainability knowledge could be included in the technical or advisory committees selected to carry out the tasks. (Schneeman)

---

*These points were made by the individual workshop speakers identified above. They are not intended to reflect a consensus among workshop speakers.

"first point of maturity." However, he observed, much of the work still revolves around national case studies, which feature widely varying reference diets, environmental footprints, and scenario designs. He emphasized that this variation complicates comparisons across studies and makes it difficult to make sense of the totality of the literature. In addition, he noted, the predominant focus with respect to environmental impact has been on greenhouse gas (GHG) emissions, and only a few studies have examined land and water use. Moreover, he said, health impacts often are not explicitly analyzed beyond adherence to national dietary guidelines or directional changes in nutrient levels (Payne et al., 2016).

A Combined Analysis of the Health and Environmental Impacts of Sustainable-Diet Strategies

Springmann went on to discuss a combined analysis of the health and environmental impacts of sustainable-diet strategies across 158 countries.

Methods: The Dietary Change Strategies Analyzed

Springmann explained that the analysis covered three different dietary change strategies and their predicted impacts by 2030.

The first strategy ("environmental objectives") was based on what many studies have revealed about the environmental impacts of animal-source foods. In a series of four scenarios, Springmann reported, the model reduced animal-based products and substituted plant-based products (two-thirds legumes and one-third fruits and vegetables) based on observational data on dietary patterns (how vegetarians change their diets compared with omnivores). The scenarios ranged from 25 percent substitution for animal-based foods to 100 percent substitution.

The second strategy ("food security objectives") addressed energy imbalances, including both underweight and overweight and obesity. Again, a series of scenarios was modeled, ranging from 25 to 100 percent reduction of energy imbalance.

The third strategy ("public health objectives") adopted nutritionally balanced dietary patterns developed by the EAT-Lancet Commission on Healthy Diets from Sustainable Food Systems and regionalized based on country-level preferences for types of grains, fruits, and meats. Springmann explained that because these dietary patterns were also energy-balanced patterns, this third strategy addressed the same energy imbalances addressed by the second strategy. Again, a range of scenarios was modeled: flexitarian, pescetarian, vegetarian, and vegan dietary patterns. Springmann pointed out that all of these patterns are predominantly plant based—even the flexitarian dietary pattern, which includes meat-based products but in amounts that are much smaller than those in an omnivore diet. For example, the flexitarian pattern that was modeled included only 100 grams of red meat per week.

Methods: The Modeling Framework

Springmann and his research team used a coupled modeling framework supporting five analyses: (1) a mortality analysis that involved a comparative risk assessment with nine dietary and weight-related risk factors and five disease endpoints based on the Oxford Global Health model (Springmann et al., 2016a,b); (2) an environmental analysis of country-specific footprints for GHG emissions, cropland use, freshwater use, nitrogen application, and phosphorous application (Springmann et al., 2018); (3) a regional analysis that entailed grouping all 158 countries by income (Robinson et al., 2015); (4) a nutritional analysis of 24 nutrients, based on the GENuS dataset (Smith et al., 2016) and USDA data (for vitamins B5 and B12), relative to World Health Organization (WHO) recommendations; and (5) an economic analysis of food expenditures based on country-specific estimates of food prices (Robinson et al., 2015).

Springmann observed that the Oxford Global Health model used to conduct the mortality analysis is similar to the modeling work of GBD. In addition, he noted that the environmental analysis was not life cycle based. He explained that there are two different ways of accounting for environmental impacts, one being to track at a very detailed level every emission from producing a food (i.e., life-cycle analysis [LCA]). Without going into detail, he mentioned only that the other method, which he and his team used, is a more mechanistic approach that he believes is arguably more comparable across regions and countries. (See Chapter 5 for additional discussion of the role of LCA in understanding the environmental impacts of a food system.)

Results: Mortality Analysis

According to Springmann, the mortality analysis revealed about a 10 percent reduction in premature mortality in 2030 with both the environmental strategy (the first strategy described above) and the food security strategy (the second strategy described above). The reduction associated with the environmental strategy was slightly larger, he noted, mainly as a result of increased vegetable consumption when animal-based products were replaced by plant-based products. With the food security strategy, most of the reduction in premature mortality resulted from reductions in obesity, followed by reductions in underweight.

Springmann went on to report that, because the public health strategy essentially doubles the health benefits of the food security strategy by balancing the nutritional composition of not only diet but also energy, the reduction in premature mortality associated with that strategy was similarly approximately double that of the food security strategy. It was also approximately double that of the environmental strategy. Rather than delving into any detail as to how the four public health strategy dietary scenarios (flexitarian, pescetarian, vegetarian, and vegan) compared with each other, Springmann wanted only to emphasize that all four scenarios were better in terms of reduced premature mortality than any of the other strategies (i.e., environmental or food security).

Results: Environmental Analysis

As with premature mortality, Springmann continued, all three strategies yielded reductions in environmental impact (see Figure 4-1). He explained that with the food security strategy, because there is a greater percentage of overweight and obese people than underweight people worldwide, correcting for energy imbalance effectively removes food from the system, and consequently the environmental impacts of that food.

With the environmental strategy, whereby animal-based products are replaced with plant-based products, "the story is a bit different," Springmann said. The removal of animal-based foods led to a very high reduction in GHG emissions, thus accounting for the overall reduced environmental impact of all four scenarios. However, because many plant-based foods use a

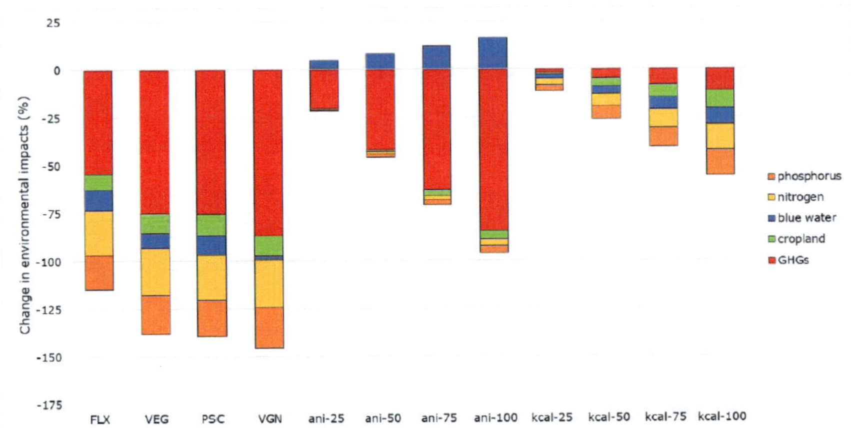

FIGURE 4-1 Environmental impacts (by 2030) of three different dietary change strategies: (1) public health strategy, (2) environmental strategy, and (3) food security strategy.
NOTES: ani-25 = 25 percent replacement of animal-based foods with plant-based foods; ani-50 = 50 percent replacement of animal-based foods with plant-based foods; ani-75 = 75 percent replacement of animal-based foods with plant-based foods; ani-100 = 100 percent replacement of animal-based foods with plant-based foods; blue water = freshwater; FLX = flexitarian diet; kcal-25 = 25 percent reduction in overweight, obesity, and underweight; kcal-50 = 50 percent reduction in overweight, obesity, and underweight; kcal-75 = 75 percent reduction in overweight, obesity, and underweight; kcal-100 = 100 percent reduction in overweight, obesity, and underweight; PSC = pescetarian diet; VEG = vegetarian diet; VGN = vegan diet. Environmental impacts include greenhouse gas (GHG) emissions, cropland use, freshwater use, nitrogen application, and phosphorous application.
SOURCE: Presented by Marco Springmann on August 1, 2018.

great deal of water, as shown in Figure 4-1, the environmental impact with respect to water use actually increased across all four dietary scenarios.

Again, Springmann reported, with the public health strategy, combining reductions in energy imbalance with a more balanced formulation of dietary intake by food group resulted in reductions in overall environmental impact much larger than those for either of the other strategies. However, some of the specific impacts, such as for water use, were not large.

Results: Regional Analysis

Springmann noted that the above results paint a global picture. He explained how grouping all 158 countries by income (high income, upper middle income, lower middle income, and low income) reveals regional specificity.

With the food security strategy, Springmann reported, all regions except low-income countries would be expected to experience small reductions in all of the measured health and environmental outcomes by 2030 (see Figure 4-2a). He interpreted these findings to mean that people in low-income countries consume too little, and that addressing energy imbalances would actually increase consumption and along with it, cropland use, GHG emissions, and freshwater use. Nitrogen and phosphorous applications, however, would be expected to decrease slightly because of future technological improvements anticipated to outweigh any increases that would otherwise occur.

In contrast, Springmann continued, with the environmental strategy scenarios, large reductions in GHG emissions occurred across all regions (see Figure 4-2b). In addition, he observed, all regions would be expected to undergo reductions in premature mortality, although those reductions would not be expected to be as large in low-income countries because these countries do not consume as many animal-based products that could be substituted for. Low-income countries would also experience a very high increase in cropland use, while all of the other regions would experience reductions. Freshwater use would increase everywhere, and the application of both nitrogen and phosphorous would increase in both low- and middle-income countries.

With a public health approach, Springmann noted, the impacts would be a little more balanced. Still, he said, "you do not get reductions everywhere. There are trade-offs." For example, with the flexitarian diet (see Figure 4-2c), all regions would see reductions in premature mortality, GHG emissions, and nitrogen application. While most regions would also see reductions in the other impacts, cropland use, freshwater use, and phosphorous application would all increase in low-income countries.

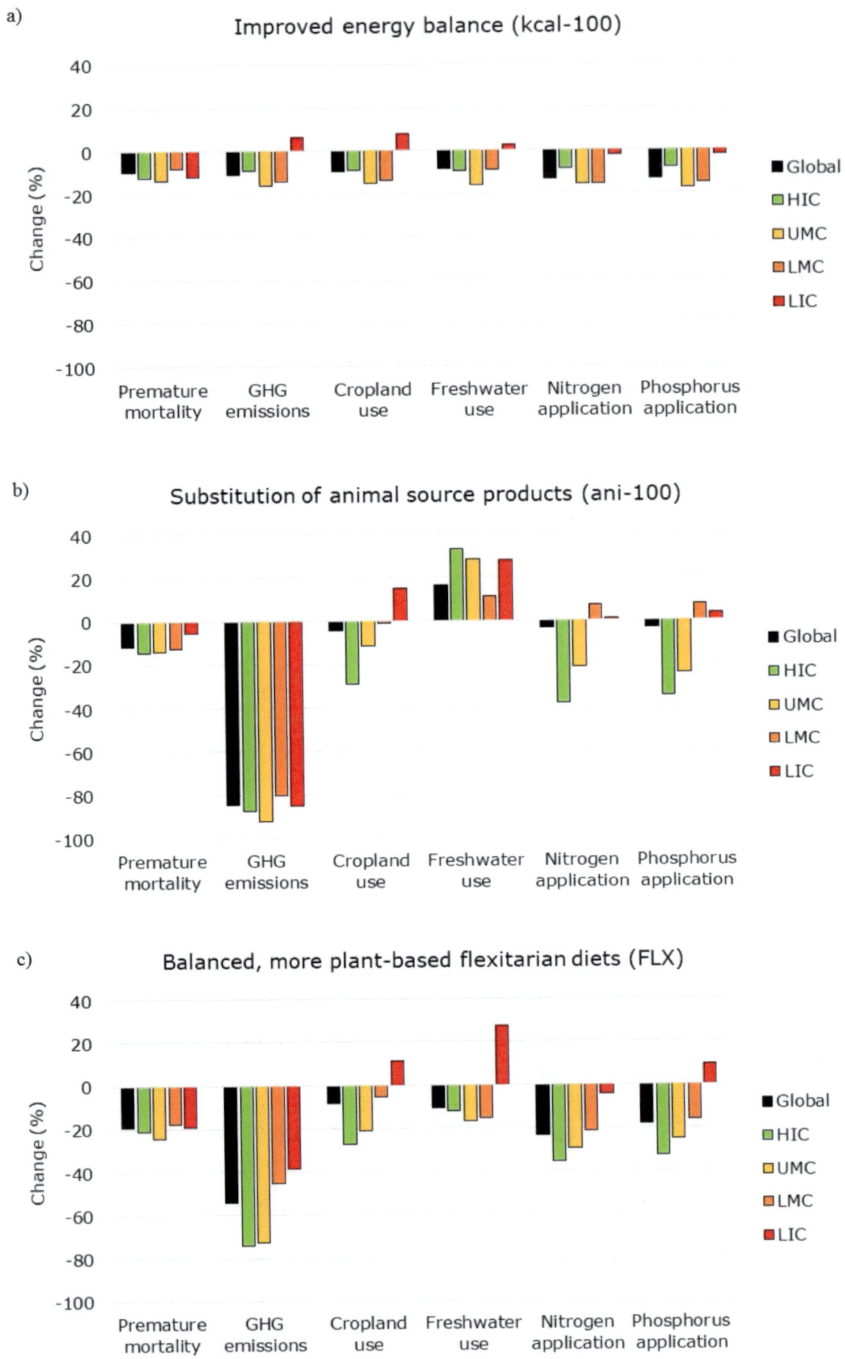
a)
Improved energy balance (kcal-100)
b)
Substitution of animal source products (ani-100)
c)
Balanced, more plant-based flexitarian diets (FLX)
Change (%)
40
20
0
-20
-40
-60
-80
-100
Premature mortality
GHG emissions
Cropland use
Freshwater use
Nitrogen application
Phosphorus application
Global
HIC
UMC
LMC
LIC

Results: Correlation Analysis

Another way to look at these same data, Springmann continued, is to draw regional correlations between the health and environmental impacts among the different diet scenarios. Doing so reveals aligned impacts (i.e., correlations are positive) in middle- and high-income countries under most of the diet scenarios. In contrast, in low-income countries, most of the correlations are negative. Springmann explained that technologies are a major factor when one is projecting food production, particularly in low-income countries. But even with projected technologies and intensified production, he said, "there is basically no way you can align [the impacts] by 2030," although by 2050, there should be greater alignment (i.e., fewer negative correlations between health and environmental impacts in low-income countries).

Results: Nutritional Analysis

Usually when people talk about the nutritional impacts of dietary change, Springmann observed, they focus on proteins. In this analysis, proteins were not a problem nutrient for the most part, with only low-income countries projected to have any deficiencies by 2030 and only by 1 to 2 percent in a couple of the diet scenarios. But in most other countries and under most other scenarios, protein should not be a problem. Without going into detail, Springmann commented that other nutrients, such as the B vitamins and calcium, would need to be supplemented in some regions under some of the scenarios.

Results: Food Expenditure Analysis

Springmann commented briefly on the food expenditure results. With the environmental strategy, weekly food expenditures would increase because fruits and vegetables are usually fairly expensive. In contrast, weekly

FIGURE 4-2 Health and environmental impacts (by 2013) of three different dietary change strategies, by region: (a) impacts of the food security strategy when 100 percent of energy imbalances (overweight, obesity, and underweight) are corrected; (b) impacts of the environmental strategy when 100 percent of animal-source products are replaced with plant-source products; and (c) impacts of the public health strategy when the current diet is replaced with a flexitarian diet.
NOTE: GHG = greenhouse gas; HIC = high-income country; kcal = kilocalories; LIC = low-income country; LMC = lower-middle-income country; UMC = upper-middle-income country.
SOURCE: Presented by Marco Springmann on August 1, 2018.

food expenditures would decrease under the food security strategy—at least globally—because people would be eating less food. With the public health strategy, people would be eating better, but also less, in all the scenarios except pescetarian; therefore, the increased price associated with greater fruit and vegetable consumption would be compensated by the reduced price associated with eating less food. Thus, again at the global level, weekly food expenditures would decrease for all the scenarios except pescetarian, because fish are very expensive. Springmann added that when countries are categorized by region, the predictions for the public health strategy differ considerably, with low-income countries experiencing large increases in weekly food expenditures under all four public health scenarios. "That is a big problem," he said.

Final Remarks

In summary, Springmann stated that improving nutrient levels and reducing diet-related premature mortality is possible in all regions of the world, but that only in high- and middle-income countries would that achievement be aligned with a reduction in environmental impacts. He called for a synergistic perspective on sustainable diets that takes account of regional considerations, including technological changes and perhaps international support mechanisms. He noted that while reducing GHG emissions is important at the global level for mitigating climate change, other environmental impacts are more context-dependent.

Among the three different dietary change strategies tested, Springmann advocates the public health strategy. A strategy that balances dietary intake and food composition could, he said, "deliver quite a bit and a way to achieve sustainable diets." However, he cautioned that currently, most national dietary guidelines do not actually reflect the evidence on healthy eating used to deduce the dietary patterns modeled in his team's analyses, incorporating no or overly lax limits for animal-source foods, particularly dairy. In this regard, he considers the *Dietary Guidelines for Americans* (DGA) to be especially problematic and they are unsupported by the evidence base. "Updating national dietary guidelines should be a priority," he concluded, if such guidelines are to reflect the latest evidence on eating for both health and environmental sustainability.

REDUCING THE CARBON FOOTPRINT WITHOUT SACRIFICING AFFORDABILITY, NUTRIENT DENSITY, AND TASTE

For Jennie Macdiarmid, University of Aberdeen, Scotland, the key challenge for sustainable diets is to combine nutritional security with measures to address climate change. Given the substantial contribution of livestock to climate change, she and her research team have demonstrated, through modeling, that it is possible to have a diet that meets all nutrient requirements, is affordable, and has as low a carbon footprint as possible (90 percent reduced). "Within reason," she said, "you can optimize just about anything." But to get that 90 percent reduction in GHG emissions, she elaborated, would require eating nothing but bran flakes, pasta, peas, a few onions, and a bit of chocolate (Macdiarmid et al., 2012). "Remember," she said, "you are putting water on your bran flakes." She emphasized that one cannot rely on modeling alone to develop sustainable diets; rather, "we have to have that human input."

For a slightly more realistic diet, Macdiarmid and her research team added what they called an "acceptable" element into the same model, entailing a diet that would be more familiar to people. Again, the researchers were able to identify a combination of foods that was nutritionally adequate; with a low carbon footprint; affordable; and, in this case, also tasty. This diet contained many more food items, including small amounts of meat and dairy. The trade-off, however, was lowering the reduction in GHG emissions from 90 percent to only 25 percent.

Like Springmann, Macdiarmid commented on the number of systematic reviews conducted since this first modeling work was done, highlighting one review in particular. Aleksandrowicz and colleagues (2016) concluded that not only do plant-based diets result in lower GHG emissions relative to animal-based diets, but, more interesting in Macdiarmid's opinion, there is a range of plant-based diets with lower GHG emissions than animal-based diets (see Figure 4-3). "We mustn't think of a vegan diet," she stressed. "There is a whole range of vegan diets that can have implications for environmental impact." She added that vegan diets are probably not what they used to be. "It used to be lentils," she said, but now, such ingredients as coconut milk are being used. She emphasized the need to think about taste, not just putting foods together.

Reducing Meat Consumption: Questions and Concerns

Macdiarmid observed that discussions on reducing consumption of animal-source foods tend to focus entirely on meat. This focus, she stated, has fueled a great deal of research, a great deal of panic, and a great deal of media attention around protein and a fear that reducing meat consumption would lead to protein deficiency. She questioned whether this is a valid concern. She explained that in a recent study on nutrition security in the United Kingdom, she and her colleagues found that, between imports and domestic production, the UK protein supply is almost twice the population-level recommended intake (grams per capita per day) (Macdiarmid et al., 2018). Even if all meat were removed from the supply chain, she noted, the country

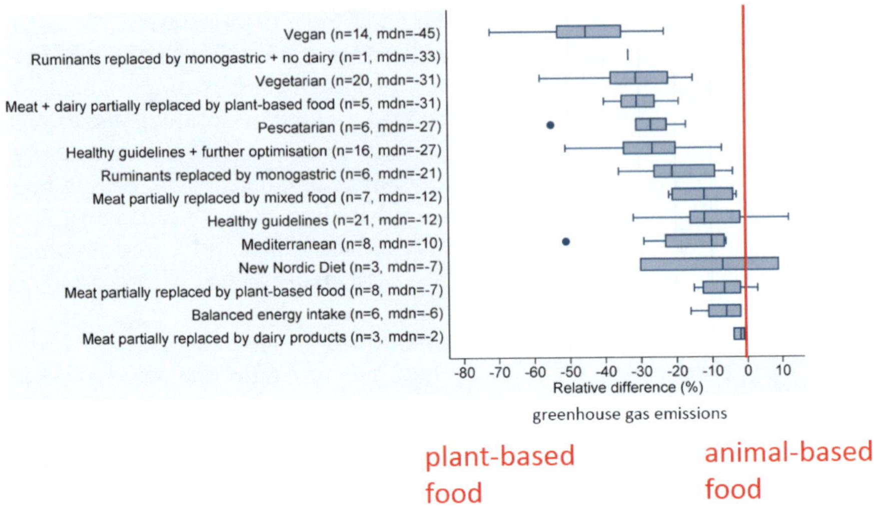

FIGURE 4-3 Range of plant-based diets associated with lower greenhouse gas emissions than animal-based diets.
SOURCES: Presented by Jennie Macdiarmid on August 1, 2018, modified from Aleksandrowicz et al., 2016.

would still have about 125 percent of its recommended protein supply. In her opinion, the attention focused on protein replacement is a distraction from other problem nutrients. She added that in all of the modeling that she and her colleagues have done, regardless of the combinations of foods they have tested (i.e., healthy and with low GHG emissions, healthy and with high GHG emissions, unhealthy and with low GHG emissions, and unhealthy and with high GHG emissions), the one outcome they have always derived is achieving the necessary amount of protein (Macdiarmid, 2013).

Macdiarmid then turned to the other issue around meat consumption—acceptability. "If we want people to change their diets," she asked, "how are we going to frame this?" This question is absolutely key, in her opinion, given that reducing meat consumption is currently not an acceptable notion, certainly not among most of the population and some governments. She cited another recent study in which her research team asked people whether they would be willing to reduce their meat consumption. Most people said no, although some said yes, and some said they would think about cutting down (Macdiarmid et al., 2016). Among those who said they would not eat less meat, reasons provided included "I like meat," "It fills me up," "I am not doing it if others will not," "It is important to me," and "Actually, it will make no difference whatsoever [to climate change]." It is because of responses like these, Macdiarmid said, that it is so important for the alternative diets being offered to be ones that people can "engage with" and are willing to eat.

Macdiarmid then alluded to the large body of research on replacing meat with legumes and various other plant-based foods. She noted as well the current trend around consumption of insects. Even in Scotland, she observed, there is a hotel that has announced it will be serving midge burgers. For her, not only does that sound unpleasant but also, and more important, insects are bioaccumulators and therefore can accumulate such contaminants as heavy metals. Thus, she highlighted the lack of debate around food safety issues associated with insects. "We need to look at the whole picture," she cautioned, "and not just say, 'This would be a good protein replacement.'" In her opinion, moreover, the insect trend is distracting from what really needs to be examined with respect to changing diets. As an example, she pointed to the low intakes of fiber in many developed countries. She suggested that this nutrient deficiency could be a more important concern than protein intake in framing the need to reduce meat and switch to a plant-based diet that would be beneficial to both health and mitigation of climate change. She added that another food being investigated is lab meat, and said she recalled a recent claim that a company had created a vegan burger that tastes exactly like meat.

Regarding the argument that reducing meat consumption could result in less costly diets, Macdiarmid remarked that whether this is true depends on what food is used to replace the meat, as well as what the resulting overall diet looks like. "We have to remember that we do not eat individual foods," she said. "We eat a collection of foods in meals and our total diet."

The Importance of Taste, Choice, and "Preswallowing" Nutrition

Although Macdiarmid agreed with others that data on sustainable diets could be refined and made more accurate (an issue that arose in the discussion at the end of the previous session, as summarized in Chapter 3), she also agreed that there are enough data and enough understanding of diets and food systems now both to improve nutrition and health and to mitigate climate change (again see Chapter 3, but also the summary of Fanzo's presentation in Chapter 2). She added that quite a bit is known about the implications of the food system for natural resources as well. But, she said, "The thing that we keep forgetting in all this discussion is around food choices. Most people do not eat just for health reasons. Most people do not eat just because they want to protect the environment." She called for a more integrated understanding of some of the factors that are actually driving what people are eating.

Macdiarmid pointed out that national dietary guidelines have existed for a long time and are often held up as evidence of accomplishments in public health nutrition. Yet, she stressed, "people still are not eating healthy diets." With respect to issuing recommendations for sustainable diets, she questioned how such recommendations would actually be implemented. She cautioned that, like national dietary guidelines, such recommendations would "get stuck" at the guideline stage absent more thought about what drives people to eat what they eat. For her, the reality that people eat for different reasons raises another key point: that everybody is different. There is no average person and there is no average diet.

Borrowing from Crotty (1993), Macdiarmid referred to the habits, desires and preferences, social influences, affordability, and other factors that drive people to make food choices—in other words, what happens before they eat—as "preswallowing nutrition." In contrast, "postswallowing" nutrition encompasses what happens biologically, or physiologically, after food is swallowed. "We focus so much on the postswallowing nutrition" and what foods do in terms of health, Macdiarmid observed, that "we have forgotten a little bit about preswallowing nutrition." Yet, she argued, preswallowing nutrition is extremely important when thinking about how to encourage people to change what they are eating.

Macdiarmid emphasized further that the context of eating varies across countries and across cultures within countries. To illustrate this point, she shared a response from a focus group study on willingness to reduce meat consumption: "I'm aware of the environment. I take other steps, I do my bit, recycling, driving less, but I probably wouldn't change diet" (Macdiarmid, 2013).

In addition to culture, Macdiarmid continued, social networks also matter. People tend to act the way people in their social networks act. In a study in which participants were asked whether they would be willing to reduce their meat consumption, one response was, "I don't want people to think I'm strange or a hippy" (Lea and Worsley, 2003).

Finally, Macdiarmid emphasized, identity influences food choice as well. "Food tells an awful lot about us," she observed. She cited a study with children who were asked to describe different foods. Boys described meat as "outgoing, popular, physically impressive, and attractive to girls," whereas girls described it as "a fat, smelly man sitting in the corner of a bar" (Elliot, 2014). She mentioned the nongovernmental organization (NGO) in the United Kingdom called Part-Time Carnivores, which found that that name attracted more men than if it were to refer to itself as being for "flexitarians" or "vegetarians." She interpreted this finding to mean that calling themselves "carnivores" gives men an identity that "flexitarian" or "vegetarian" does not. "These sorts of social things are really important to think about," she stressed.

Also important, Macdiarmid continued, is thinking about how people behave in different settings. She cited a study done a number of years ago replicating some of the work of John de Castro,[1] which showed that the amount of food people eat varies depending on the people, the number of people with whom they are eating, and where they are eating.[2] When eating with family or friends, people tend to eat more than when eating with work colleagues, she reported, and when eating in a restaurant, people tend to eat more calories than when eating at home.

Final Remarks

In summary, Macdiarmid reiterated that it is possible to model an ideal diet. She cautioned, however, that "leaving a computer to come up with it" will not necessarily lead to the change needed to achieve a sustainable diet. Rather, she argued, one should consider eating habits and behavior. She underscored the need to think about what can be done to get people to change their diets. In addition, she highlighted the need to remember that there is no such thing as an average diet. Without providing details, she briefly mentioned work of her research team showing that there are many different ways in which people can change their diet to achieve nutrient requirements while also reducing GHG emissions, and that the optimal way varies among individuals.

Finally, Macdiarmid highlighted the need to think of the food system not as a linear process but as one with many feedback loops. She emphasized that consumption is a product not just of processing and distribution but also of acceptability, preferences, the nutrition transition, cultural and social factors, and economic access.

A MENU OF SOLUTIONS FOR A SUSTAINABLE FOOD FUTURE

Building on Macdiarmid's call to better understand what drives people to make dietary choices, Janet Ranganathan, World Resources Institute (WRI), Washington, DC, discussed lessons learned from the private sector about how to shift behavior. First, however, drawing on the WRI report *Creating a Sustainable Food Future*,[3] she posed the question of how the world can feed nearly 10 billion people in 2050 in a manner that advances development and well-being while reducing pressure on the environment. "This is the question," she asserted, not just for this workshop, but for

[1]For more information, see de Castro (2000).

[2]Personal communication, S. Whybrow, European Congress of Obesity Conference, 2009.

[3]Final version forthcoming. Published installments can be viewed on the WRI website: https://www.wri.org/our-work/project/world-resources-report/world-resources-report-creating-sustainable-food-future (accessed December 18, 2018).

humanity. She has worked on almost every environmental issue during her 23 years at WRI, and every issue—from deforestation, to climate change, to eutrophication, to biodiversity—always comes back to food. Food, she said, is "the mother of all sustainability issues."

Ranganathan explained how addressing this question requires balancing three needs. First, the world needs to close the 56 percent calorie gap between 2010 and 2050, that is, the 56 percent increase in calories that WRI has predicted will be needed to feed 9.8 billion people by the latter year. According to Ranganathan, WRI predicted this gap even while assuming an additional 540 billion hectares of agricultural land and large yield improvements on par with what occurred with the green revolution. (WRI's calorie gap analysis was based on Alexandratos and Bruinsma [2012]; Bruinsma [2009]; FAO [2017a]; and UNDESA [2017].)

Second, Ranganathan observed, given that 28 percent of the world's people are employed in agriculture but that agriculture represents only about 3 percent of gross domestic product (GDP) globally (according to World Bank data) and about 1 percent in the United States, the incomes of farm workers are low. Yet, she stressed, the world needs agriculture to support economic development. She mentioned just having attended a Farmer Income Lab addressing the problem that farmers in the food company supply chains that end in developing countries are not making a living wage, adding that this explains in part why many of these people are moving to cities. She asserted that this low-income problem needs to be addressed as well while closing the calorie gap.

Third, Ranganathan identified the need for the world to reduce agriculture's impact on the environment. Currently, she observed, WRI analysis indicates that about one-quarter of the world's GHG emissions are due to agriculture when land use change is taken into account. In addition, 37 percent of the Earth's landmass (excluding Antarctica) is devoted to food production. Ranganathan pointed out that, just within her own lifetime, the agricultural footprint has expanded by about 500 million hectares, or about 60 percent of the size of the contiguous United States. "We cannot keep doing that," she stressed. Water withdrawal is a serious issue as well, she added. (WRI's environmental impact analysis was based on EIA [2012]; EPA [2012]; FAO [2011, 2012a]; Foley et al. [2005]; Houghton [2008]; IEA [2012]; and Lindquist et al. [2012].)

Production Versus Consumption Strategies for Sustainably Closing the Food Gap

According to Ranganathan, WRI recognizes that there is no "silver bullet" for meeting the above needs. She asserted that, although dietary shift may be a "shinier silver bullet" than many of the others, "we need all solutions on the table," including strategies for increasing production sustainably and other strategies for reducing growth in consumption (see Figure 4-4). Building on what several previous speakers had mentioned, she briefly described several examples of both types of strategies.

Increasing Production

According to Ranganathan, sustainable production solutions include, first, sustainably boosting yields through crop breeding. She called attention to "the other GM," meaning Gregory Mendel and classical breeding, and highlighted the potential of modern genomics to accelerate conventional crop breeding. In addition, she stressed, there are significant opportunities to increase the productivity of orphan crops, which cover large portions of land, particularly where poor farmers live.

As a second production strategy, Ranganathan pointed to improving soil and water management. As examples, she cited bringing forests back into agricultural systems and rainwater harvesting.

The third production strategy identified by Ranganathan is restoring degraded land and using it to produce food. Depending on one's definition of degraded land, there may be 1 billion hectares of degraded lands globally, she observed.

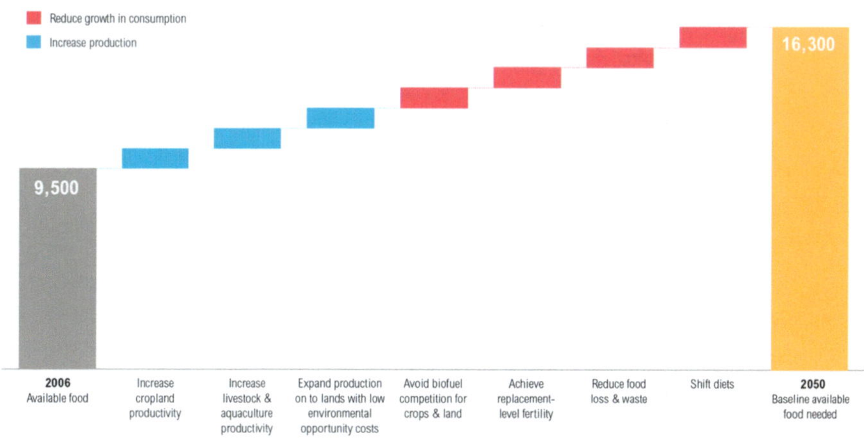

FIGURE 4-4 Range of solutions available for closing the food gap between now and 2050.
NOTE: Values depicted by bars are global crop production in trillions of kilocalories.
SOURCES: Presented by Janet Ranganathan on August 1, 2018; Ranganathan et al., 2016.

In addition to boosting crop yields, Ranganathan continued, another set of solutions pertains to sustainably increasing livestock productivity. Even though most of the research on intensification has focused on crops, she pointed out, about twice as much land is devoted to livestock production. In her view, there are many promising opportunities to increase both pastureland and livestock productivity—especially with ruminants, and beef in particular—not necessarily in the United States but in developing countries. The same is true, she suggested, for wild fish. While she acknowledged that wild fish catch will probably have to be reduced to allow overexploited fisheries to recover, there are again, she argued, good opportunities to increase the productivity and sustainability of aquaculture.

Reducing Consumption

According to Ranganathan, strategies for reducing consumption include, first, as previous speakers had mentioned, reducing food loss and waste. She noted that globally, about one-third of food by weight and about one-quarter of food by calories is lost between farm and fork. She reported that WRI is developing a protocol for measuring food loss and waste, based on the premise that "what gets measured gets managed." In addition, the Institute is building a coalition of leaders who have made commitments to reducing food loss and waste by 50 percent by 2030 and to sharing lessons learned. Known as Champion 12.3 (named after the Sustainable Development Goal and target devoted to reducing food waste), the coalition includes leaders and heads of supermarkets, companies, states, and countries. Ranganathan observed that if food waste were a country, it would rank third in GHG emissions behind China and the United States. "Just think about that," she said. "It is wasted water. It is wasted land. It is wasted greenhouse gas emissions. And it is wasted money. We have to get on that one."

Ranganathan identified as a second consumption strategy achieving replacement-level fertility. She sees this as an important opportunity in sub-Saharan Africa in particular, where the fertility rate has been about 5 births per woman over the past 5 years and is predicted to drop to about 3.2 by 2050. "We can speed that up," she argued, by doing things that should be done regardless, such as keeping girls in school, providing access to reproductive health services, and reducing infant and child mortality.

Another consumption strategy cited by Ranganathan is reducing demand for biofuel crops. She pointed out that a target of 20 percent biofuel in the energy system by 2050, an actual target in some countries, would require almost the entire biomass harvest of 2000. "Think about the extraordinary potential for competition that would create between food and fuel," she observed. "That is something we must deal with." (See Chapter 3 for a summary of Wilde's discussion of biofuel and its influence on prices.)

Finally, Ranganathan highlighted shifting diets as another consumption strategy for achieving a sustainable food future, as Springmann and others had discussed. She noted that animal-based foods are generally more land-, water-, and GHG-intensive to produce relative to plant-based foods. For every food calorie generated, she elaborated, ruminant meat requires more feed and land input and emits far greater amounts of GHGs compared with other foods. According to Ranganathan, efforts to date to shift diets have focused on education, information, and abstinence. While she believes that these approaches are important, she asserted that they are not enough. She spent the remainder of her talk discussing what WRI has learned from the private sector about shifting behavior, as summarized below.

Later, during the discussion period, Ranganathan clarified that while she was not convinced that information provided in the DGA directly influences what foods people order or buy, she believes it does in fact have a significant influence on the food manufacturing and food services sectors.

Strategies for Shifting Diet: Lessons from the Private Sector

"The private sector knows how to influence people's consumption choices," Ranganathan said. Rather than examining how taxes, subsidies, and other governmental mechanisms can influence people's food choices, WRI chose to examine how the private sector uses marketing and behavioral science to influence people's choices.

Four Common Strategies

In an analysis of more than 20 successful consumption shifts that have already occurred in the consumer goods sector, Ranganathan and colleagues identified four common strategies that work in concert.

The first is to minimize disruption. According to Ranganathan, this is what companies marketing fake meat are trying to do by providing something that looks like regular meat and can be barbequed or otherwise prepared like regular meat. This is also why some merchants place soy milk in the refrigerated section of the market where people habitually go to get their milk, even though soy milk does not need to be refrigerated.

The second strategy is to sell a compelling benefit. In other words, Ranganathan explained, do not tell people why a product is good for them or bad for the environment and hope that they will shift to something else. Rather, think about what consumers actually want, such as taste and affordability.

The third strategy is to maximize awareness, which Ranganathan characterized as "a tried and tested strategy by the private sector." The products marketers want to sell the most, for example, are placed at the end of an aisle in a supermarket or at the top of a menu in a restaurant. Things they do not want consumers to purchase because those products have a lower profit margin are placed on lower supermarket shelves.

Fourth is evolving norms. Ranganathan cited just one example: "If you think about the last time you saw a man in public cooking food, he was probably cooking a beef burger on a barbeque." She referred to Macdiarmid's earlier discussion of other examples of social norms and encouraged more thinking about how to evolve them to favor more sustainable food choices, such as plant-based rather than animal-based food.

Case Study: Low-Alcohol Beer

Around 2000, the UK government stated that it wanted to remove 1 billion units of alcohol from the market, out of concern about binge drinking and alcoholism. Thus, Ranganathan explained, the government challenged the beverage sector to help shift consumers from drinking beverages with high to those with low alcohol content. She recounted how Molson, which makes Carling, accepted the challenge because it had a low-alcohol alternative and did not want to lose market share. But the company faced a number of barriers, she observed: people did not want low-alcohol beer, they did not like the taste of it, and it was usually located in the low-traffic, "low-alcohol" section of supermarkets. To get around these barriers, Ranganathan explained, Molson took a number of actions, all of which aligned with those presented in WRI's shift wheel (see Figure 4-5): it masked the bitter taste by creating ginger and lime flavors (i.e., it minimized disruption by disguising the change); it positioned the new product around the benefit of a lower-carb refreshment, making no mention of its alcohol content (i.e., it sold a compelling benefit); and it gave the product a new name, Carling Zest. At the same time, Ranganathan added, the UK government increased the excise tax on high-alcohol drinks and reduced it on low-alcohol beer, so the price of the new product went down. Instead of passing that savings on to consumers, Molson passed it on to retailers, increasing the profit margin from selling this brand, thus incentivizing the retailers to give Carling Zest a more prominent shelf space (i.e., maximizing awareness). As a result of these actions, according to Ranganathan, this was a successful rebranding campaign.

Ranganathan described how Unilever did much the same thing to shift people from cod-based to pollock-based fish fingers, that is, from an overfished to a more prevalent species, and in the process to reduce its raw material costs. The barriers to this strategy, Ranganathan observed, were a strong association between fish fingers and cod; an assumption that pollock does not taste as good as cod; and the gray, not white, color of pollock, which was off-putting to consumers. She explained that by positioning

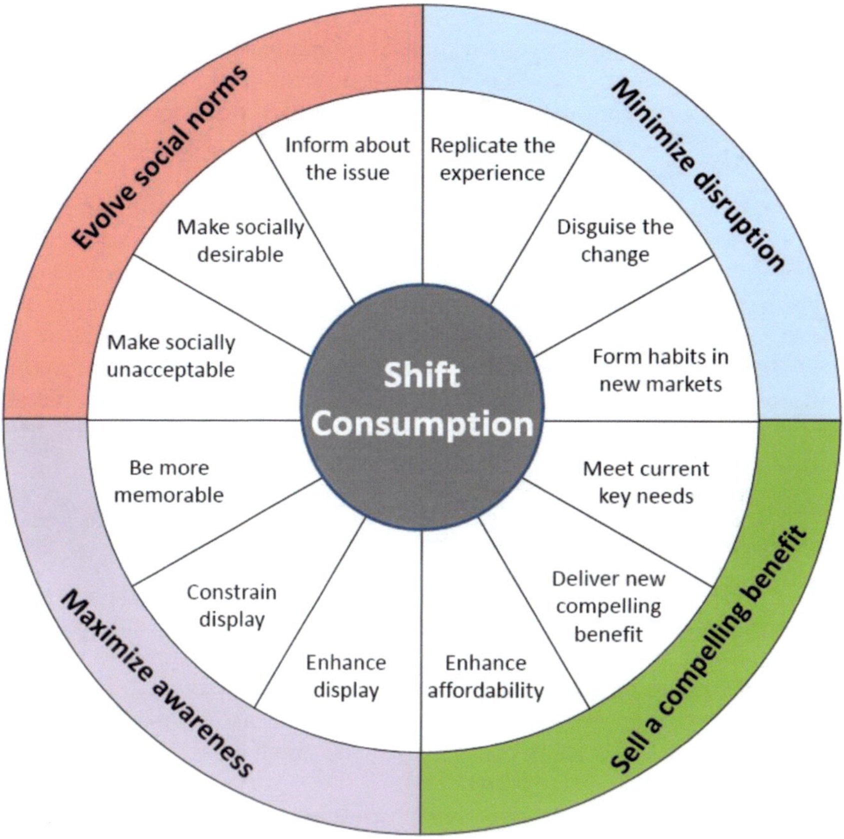

FIGURE 4-5 A "shift wheel" with four common strategies for shifting consumer behavior (outer ring) and key features of each strategy (wedges).
SOURCES: Presented by Janet Ranganathan on August 1, 2018, modified from Ranganathan et al., 2016.

the pollock-based product around the health benefit of its higher omega-3 content (i.e., selling a compelling benefit) and by passing on some of the savings in raw material costs to retailers, the company encouraged retailers to promote and display the new fish fingers (i.e., maximizing awareness).

Strategies for Shifting Diet: Lessons from the Food Services Sector

In addition to its study of the retail sector, Ranganathan continued, WRI has been studying consumer behavior in the food services sector. She argued that, with respect to encouraging consumers to choose more plant-based foods, the food services sector may be an easier target than the retail sector for three reasons. First, she observed, in the United States, as much money is spent on food consumed outside as inside the home. Second, she pointed out that the incentives of the food services sector are aligned with the objective of shifting diets because it sells meals, not foods. Third, she noted that habits formed outside the home are often brought back into the home.

Ranganathan reported that WRI created its Better Buying Lab with a group of food service companies to experiment with ways of shifting food choices in the United States and the United Kingdom. She explained that the lab generates ideas, tests those ideas with the food service companies, and then shares more broadly what has been learned. Currently, she said, the lab is focused on three areas: (1) transforming how the food industry communicates about plant-based foods, (2) popularizing dishes rich in plants, and (3) identifying the right environmental targets and metrics. She then discussed the first two of these efforts in more detail.

Language and Framing: Transforming How the Food Industry Communicates About Plant-Based Foods

Ranganathan asked workshop participants to imagine being presented at a restaurant with a menu containing an entrée described as "baked squash with rice and grits." Then, she asked them to imagine being presented with a menu describing that same entrée as "roasted butternut squash with sweet and spicy coconut rice and fresh Thai basil." Which is more attractive to you? she asked.

It is not just language but also positioning on a menu that can be used to shift behavior, Ranganathan continued. She described a study that WRI conducted in collaboration with the London School of Economics that involved comparing menus containing a separate box for vegetarian dishes ("vegetarian" menu) with menus in which vegetarian dishes were included in the main section of the menu ("control" menu). She reported that, among 760 study participants in the United Kingdom, 13.4 percent ordered vegetarian entrées from the control menu, compared with only 5.9 percent who ordered from the vegetarian menu (Bacon and Krpan, 2018).

Ranganathan described another study, not conducted by the Better Buying Lab, in which researchers compared four ways of framing the same vegetable: indulgent (e.g., "twisted garlic ginger butternut squash wedges"), basic ("butternut squash"), healthy restrictive ("butternut squash with no added sugar"), and healthy positive ("antioxidant-rich butternut squash") (Turnwald et al., 2017). The study revealed that using indulgent language resulted in significantly more people selecting a vegetable relative to when that same vegetable was described using either basic, healthy restrictive, or healthy positive language. "Language, I think, does matter," Ranganathan concluded. At the same time, however, she cautioned against overselling this claim, and she described this as a nascent but fertile research area.

Power Dishes: Popularizing Dishes Rich in Plants

A second strategy being tested at the Better Buying Lab is to popularize dishes rich in plants by increasing the number of plant-based "power dishes," defined as dishes that are prevalent on menus in mainstream restaurants. Currently, Ranganathan reported, only one vegetarian dish—the ubiquitous "veggie sandwich/wrap"—is among the top 25 most prevalent dishes on menus in U.S. restaurants. She described how the lab has been working on introducing three additional vegetarian power dishes: a blended burger (30 percent mushroom, 70 percent beef), a veggie bowl, and an avocado club sandwich. Given that 1 billion beef burgers are sold in the United States annually, she observed, even if only 30 percent of the beef in each of those burgers was replaced with mushrooms, in terms of GHG emissions that would be like taking 2.3 million cars, or about the total number of cars in San Diego, off U.S. roads.

Supply Chain Greenhouse Gas Emissions

In closing, Ranganathan mentioned briefly that while many food service companies have made commitments to GHG reduction, most of their efforts are centered around transportation and energy. She stated that WRI is also working to encourage them to think about the GHG emissions resulting from their food supply chains. She observed that shifting consumers to more plant-based foods can be an effective GHG reduction strategy as well.

THE CASE FOR NUTRITION-SENSITIVE VALUE CHAIN INTERVENTIONS: WHAT GETS MEASURED GETS IMPROVED

While most of the workshop discussion on actions that can support sustainable diets revolved around production versus consumption strategies, Maha Tahiri, former food industry executive, addressed the challenges and opportunities for achieving sustainable diets through a different lens: nutrition-sensitive value chain (NSVC) interventions. Referring back to Fanzo's earlier remarks about policy making (see Chapter 2), she suggested that NSVCs are something policy makers and the private sector should take into account.

Historically, Tahiri observed, most food chain interventions have been aimed at increasing yield and the well-being of farmers. She explained how the concept of an NSVC, with its focus on nutritional outcomes, not just economic value, emerged about 10 years ago based on the premise that "what gets measured gets improved." She noted that, in the NSVC

BOX 4-2
Definition of a Nutrition-Sensitive Value Chain

"Nutrition-sensitive value chain—A food value chain consists of all the stakeholders who participate in the coordinated production and value-adding activities that are needed to make food products (FAO, 2014). Though the traditional focus has been on economic value, nutrition-sensitive value chains leverage opportunities to enhance supply and/or demand for nutritious food, as well as opportunities to add nutritional value (and/or minimize food and nutrient loss) at each step of the chain, thereby improving the availability, affordability, quality, and acceptability of nutritious food. For lasting impacts on nutrition, this approach must be placed in a sustainability context as well."

SOURCE: FAO, 2017b.

definition articulated by an FAO-hosted Rome-based Agencies[4] working group on NSVCs (FAO, 2017b; see Box 4-2), she was particularly struck by its focus on the whole value chain, from input, through preparation, to consumption.

Rationale for the NSVC Approach

Tahiri called attention to a handful of studies reporting that traditional interventions, such as food fortification, complementary feeding, and promotion of breastfeeding, are not enough to achieve global nutrition targets. First, she pointed to a study conducted by *The Lancet*'s Maternal and Child Undernutrition Group as being particularly important (Bhutta et al., 2008). Among 36 countries representing 90 percent of the global malnutrition burden, the researchers concluded that implementation of evidence-based interventions would not achieve global targets. Tahiri then cited a follow-up study in which Bhutta and colleagues (2013) demonstrated that implementing 10 evidence-based nutrition-specific interventions, including breastfeeding, fortification, and community interventions, with 90 percent coverage would reduce deaths among children younger than 5 years by only 15 percent and reduce stunting by only 20 percent. The authors concluded that nutrition interventions should be combined with nutrition-sensitive approaches that address the underlying determinants of malnutrition, such as women's empowerment, education, employment, social protection, and

[4]The Rome-based agencies include FAO, the International Fund for Agricultural Development (IFAD), the World Food Programme (WFP), and the Bioversity International.

safety nets. Lastly, Tahiri highlighted a review paper on the impacts of agriculture on nutrition (Webb and Kennedy, 2014), in which the authors analyze 10 well-implemented interventions and conclude that the "empirical evidence for plausible and significant impacts of agriculture on defined nutrition outcomes remains disappointingly scarce." Tahiri pointed out, however, as the authors do, that the absence of evidence is not the same as evidence of absence. Agriculture and nutrition are both very large domains, she explained, and unless an analysis is more specific, it makes sense that significant correlations would not be detected.

Strategies for NSVC Intervention

Tahiri identified as one particularly positive feature of NSVCs that they make it possible to divide the complex food system into different parts and visualize, depending on the situation (i.e., increased demand versus increased supply), how an intervention at any point along the value chain could enhance nutrition (see Figure 4-6). In this way, she posited, they help people formulate questions in a more expansive way, including how to act in the interest of sustainability.

As an example of a possible NSVC intervention in a situation of high demand and inconsistent supply, Tahiri mentioned labor-saving methods at the input stage, which would also have sustainability implications in the sense that such a strategy would mean more time for mothers to care for their children. She cited refrigerated transport at the distribution/transport stage as another example of an NSVC intervention in such a situation that would also have implications for sustainability. In contrast, in a situation of

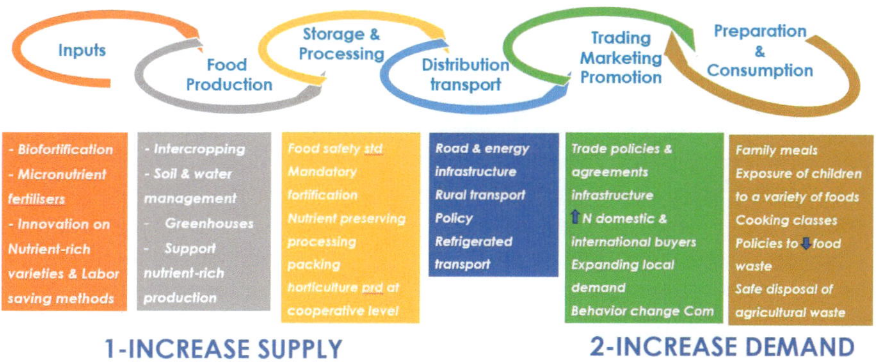

FIGURE 4-6 Strategies for nutrition-sensitive value chain interventions.
NOTE: N = population; prd = product; std = standard.
SOURCES: Presented by Maha Tahiri on August 1, 2018, modified from FAO, 2017b.

high demand and consistent supply, she suggested that the focus probably should be on food safety. In a situation of demand constraint and consistent supply, she stated that interventions would be targeted at the trading/marketing/promotion stage of the value chain. Finally, she observed that in a situation of demand constraint and inconsistent supply, interventions would probably need to be applied all along the chain.

NSVC Interventions: An Example and Proof of Concept

As an example of an NSVC, Tahiri described work conducted by the International Food Policy Research Institute (IFPRI) in Rwanda and Uganda to increase the availability of, access to, and demand for nutritious beans (Mazur et al., 2009). She noted that beans are very important in both countries. She reported that the researchers conducted field trials with new varieties of beans, training farmers on the spacing of rows and other production techniques. They also trained farmers on anaerobic storage and other postharvest technologies. In addition, they worked with the farmers to help them understand the market and to sell their beans collectively. Tahiri pointed out that when the farmers sold individually, only about 10 percent would actually sell their beans on any given day, whereas when they sold collectively, more than 81 percent were able to sell their beans. Finally, Tahiri said, the researchers also worked with the farmers to improve their negotiation skills and increase demand from other countries, namely South Sudan and Kenya. In sum, she explained, they examined all aspects of the value chain to see where they could make improvements. However, she cautioned, this was not a controlled study, so it was not possible to say that the interventions were any more effective than traditional interventions.

Tahiri said she was unaware of any controlled studies of NSVC interventions. What she characterized as the "best" she could find was what she considers a proof-of-concept study conducted in North Senegal (Le Port et al., 2017). She described how this study involved a value chain that already existed—a local dairy factory, Laiterie du Berger—that had been receiving milk from its network of seminomadic, pastoralist dairy farmers, but on an irregular basis. Tahiri explained that the intervention involved a year-long exchange between the farmers and the factory, whereby the farmers delivered a constant supply of milk to the factory 5 days per week in return for a fortified yogurt produced from that milk that the farmers would then feed to their children. She added that the study was conducted while a behavioral change communication campaign related to fortified products was being implemented nationwide. The researchers found that after 1 year, the prevalence of anemia among children aged 24 to 59 months had declined from 80 percent to 60 percent. The impact was greater on boys than on girls. Although this was not a case-control study, Tahiri said, it was "what

I would say is really good proof of concept of a nutrition-sensitive value chain intervention."

Final Remarks

Tahiri concluded by highlighting what she considers to be key factors in the success of NSVC interventions. She identified as one of the most important that there be a clear definition of the nutrition problem, and therefore of the nutrition goal. In addition, she called for an expansive search for creative solutions that can be applied locally. Next, she highlighted coordination of the whole chain as key, although she acknowledged that this sometimes is not possible; for example, when no transportation is available.

Tahiri cited adding value to all actors along the value chain as another key factor driving success and as one of the keys to the success of the North Senegal dairy intervention: Laiterie du Berger received a constant supply of milk, and the herders received a fortified yogurt for their children. Referring to the philanthropic work done by many companies in Africa, India, and elsewhere, she pointed out that "all actors along the value chain" include the private sector. She encouraged more engagement of the private sector—from large, vertically integrated, multinational companies to individuals who transport, store, aggregate, or sell food.

Yet another key factor in success, Tahiri stressed, is to adopt a "consumer first" approach, which she believes is the best way to increase or create demand. Even when people say they want to have sustainable products, she noted, consumer research has shown that when consumers are actually making a purchase, they do not buy a product unless there is something specific and "close to home" about it that they can embrace.

Finally, Tahiri underscored the need to focus on influencing policy. Specifically, she pointed to the importance of elevating nutrition in the agenda.

OPPORTUNITIES FOR INTEGRATING SUSTAINABILITY AND DIETARY GUIDANCE

Barbara Schneeman, University of California, Davis, who served on a National Academies committee examining the process for establishing the DGA (NASEM, 2017), addressed how sustainability could be integrated into the DGA. She used that committee's report, *Redesigning the Process for Establishing the* Dietary Guidelines for Americans, as the basis for her presentation. She characterized it as particularly useful for this purpose because the committee did such a thorough job of examining the evolution of the DGA and the methodology used to establish the guidelines. The committee, she explained, identified three essential functions, or phases, currently carried out by the Dietary Guidelines Advisory Committee (DGAC), working in collaboration with staff from the U.S. Department of Health and Human Services (HHS) and USDA: (1) strategic planning, (2) analysis, and (3) synthesis/interpretation. Schneeman did not think it necessary, for the purposes of this talk, to go into detail on the redesign of the DGA cycle proposed by the National Academies committee (i.e., a 5-year cycle between releases of subsequent DGAs). She did emphasize, however, the committee's recognition that each phase requires the right expertise and right investment of time and resources. Therefore, she reported, the committee proposed that different DGA committees be responsible for each of the three essential phases. Schneeman went on to consider how sustainability could be integrated into each of these phases through the work of the proposed DGA committees and in other ways.

Integrating Sustainability into *Dietary Guidelines for Americans* Strategic Planning

In general, the National Academies committee encouraged more strategic planning across DGA cycles and a longer-term look at development of the guidelines. Specifically, the committee proposed that a Planning and Continuity Group "provide the secretaries of USDA and HHS with planning support that assures alignment with long-term strategic objectives spanning multiple DGA cycles, identify and prioritize topics for the [Dietary Guidelines Scientific Advisory Committee] to evaluate in subsequent DGA cycles, and oversee monitoring and surveillance for new evidence." Schneeman clarified that this planning group would not be involved with developing or evaluating evidence, but with determining whether there is evidence suggesting that a topic might be "ready for prime time."

In the context of how sustainability might be integrated into the strategic planning phase, Schneeman identified two key opportunities: first, determining how sustainability relates to the purpose of the DGA, and second, delineating sustainability topics to be addressed in subsequent cycles.

Determining How Sustainability Relates to the Purpose of the Dietary Guidelines for Americans

The National Academies committee identified multiple statements about the purpose of and audience for the DGA, Schneeman reported, leading it to urge continuity and clarity around these statements. In fact, she said, the committee proposed a singular purpose statement aligned with wording in the legislation that established the DGA cycle (i.e., the National Nutrition Monitoring and Related Research Act): "The purpose of the DGA is to provide science-based 'nutritional and dietary information and guidelines for the general public' that form the basis for 'any federal food, nutrition, or health program.'" Schneeman added that the committee proposed that the audience for the DGA be the general public and that the goals of the guidelines be to promote dietary intake that helps improve health and reduce the risk of chronic disease and to provide the federal government with a consistent approach for nutrition policy and messaging. Although sustainability is not an explicit part of the proposed purpose statement, she asserted that there would be ways to accomplish this.

Delineating Sustainability Topics to Be Addressed

Regarding the identification and prioritization of topics to be evaluated during subsequent DGA cycles, Schneeman continued, the National Academies committee divided criteria for topic selection into three categories: topic identification, topic selection, and topic prioritization. She explained that the first two categories are areas in which there probably should be nongovernmental stakeholder as well as government input. In contrast, the committee identified topic prioritization as a task for the proposed Planning and Continuity Group. As with the purpose statement, Schneeman added, sustainability was not incorporated as an explicit criterion for any of the three categories of criteria. Criteria for topic identification, she elaborated, focus more on relevance to diet, nutrition, and health. While the criteria for prioritization suggest cost-effectiveness studies, their focus is more on public health urgency and the availability of evidence-based intervention. In Schneeman's opinion, again, there clearly is an opportunity to consider how sustainability could be integrated into this scheme. She mentioned that HHS and USDA asked for comments on topics during the last DGA cycle, so there does appear to be some interest in opening the process up to suggestions. However, she was unaware of whether any sustainability-related topics were advanced. She stressed that in the future, depending on the topic(s) chosen, the relevant expertise will need to be brought to bear, either through membership of the Planning and Continuity Group or through any subcommittees that are formed. Either way, she said, "that expertise needs to be part of the process."

Challenges to Integrating Sustainability into Dietary Guidelines for Americans *Strategic Planning*

In Schneeman's opinion, integrating sustainability into DGA strategic planning presents an opportunity, but also challenges. She identified as a key challenge understanding the objective for incorporating sustainability. Is it to justify the recommendations? Is it to consider the environmental impacts of dietary shifts? Or is it to see whether the recommendations are feasible given current economic and agricultural capacity? Schneeman observed that all of these questions had been touched on during this workshop. In addition, she pointed to a 1998 WHO/FAO report, *Preparation and Use of Food-Based Dietary Guidelines*, which emphasizes the importance of addressing such issues as economic and agricultural capacity when developing food-based dietary guidelines (WHO and FAO, 1998).

Integrating Sustainability into *Dietary Guidelines for Americans* Analysis

According to Schneeman, the types of evidence currently used to develop the DGA include original systematic reviews conducted with support from USDA's Nutrition Evidence Library (NEL); existing systematic reviews, meta-analyses, and reports that are relevant and that meet the process criteria; descriptive data analyses, such as intakes of food and nutrients (e.g., from the National Health and Nutrition Examination Survey's [NHANES's] *What We Eat in America*); and, increasingly, food pattern modeling analyses aimed at determining what kind of food patterns meet the DGA recommendations. The National Academies committee proposed the use of technical expert panels (TEPs) to provide independent expertise during the analysis phase. Schneeman explained that a TEP could be assembled to help with systematic reviews, or if there were a specialized topic relating to a certain aspect of sustainability, a TEP could be assembled to assist with the technical review of that topic. In Schneeman's opinion, supplemental expertise in food pattern modeling and descriptive data analysis could become critical if sustainability were incorporated as a factor.

In Schneeman's opinion, probably the most important challenges to integrating sustainability into the analysis phase of the cycle are defining the topics and research questions that can be addressed with systematic reviews and identifying the descriptive data analyses that are most relevant. As she had mentioned previously, the NHANES is one of the primary sources currently used for descriptive data analysis. But what is the most relevant tool from a sustainability point of view?, Schneeman asked. And how should food pattern modeling be considered in relation to sustainability? Given that food pattern modeling is used to see what patterns meet the DGA recommendations, does sustainability now need to be built into the way these models are constructed? Again, Schneeman stressed, the TEPs would need to include experts with knowledge in these areas.

Integrating Sustainability into *Dietary Guidelines for Americans* Synthesis and Interpretation

Schneeman observed that work conducted during the third phase, synthesis and interpretation, is what most people associate with the current DGAC. She noted that the National Academies committee proposed renaming the DGAC the Dietary Guidelines Scientific Advisory Committee (DGSAC) to emphasize the science, as it is during this phase that the DGAC synthesizes, interprets, and integrates the data and evidence across studies to develop conclusions and recommendations. In addition, the DGAC identifies new analyses that might be needed, topics on which more evidence is needed, and topics for future DGA cycles, as well as research recommendations. The main task, though, according to Schneeman, is to produce a scientific report for the secretaries of HHS and USDA to serve as a foundation for the DGA Policy Report.

Schneeman explained that integrating sustainability into this third phase would involve, again, including experts who can provide relevant knowledge and context for a review of the evidence on topics identified as relevant for consideration in the DGA. She noted the report of the National Academies committee (NASEM, 2017) refers to an earlier report on the selection process for DGAC members, and she pointed out that those same criteria would have to be applied to the selection of sustainability experts for the DGAC (or the renamed DGSAC).

The main challenge to integrating sustainability into the DGA synthesis and interpretation phase, as Schneeman sees it, is that the process for nominating and selecting DGAC (DGSAC) members with the relevant sustainability expertise would depend on having identified specific areas of sustainability to be considered in that cycle.

Final Remarks

The opportunities discussed by Schneeman for integrating sustainability into the three key phases of the DGA process are summarized in Table 4-1. She noted that she had not discussed the final phase, federal review and update, which is what leads to publication of the DGA Policy Report. In her opinion, if there is transparency in the three earlier phases regarding the integration of relevant sustainability topics, this final phase "takes care of itself."

Schneeman's take-home message was that to integrate sustainability into the DGA, it will be necessary to clarify the relationship between sustainability and the purpose of the DGA. Another key challenge, she suggested, will be to reexamine the resources for the three phases (strategic planning, analysis, and synthesis/interpretation) to see how they might need to be shifted so that sustainability can be addressed.

Finally, Schneeman mentioned that one of the recommendations of the National Academies committee was to consider the emerging importance of systems approaches. Specifically, recommendation 7 of the committee's report (NASEM, 2017) was: "The secretaries of USDA and HHS should commission research and evaluate strategies to develop and implement

TABLE 4-1 Opportunities to Integrate Sustainability into the Different Phases of the National Academies' Proposed *Dietary Guidelines for Americans* Process

Phase	Opportunities
Strategic Planning	• Clarify the role of sustainability in the purpose of the DGA; • Identify the topics and objectives related to sustainability that are relevant to the DGA; and • Develop a long-term plan for addressing sustainability across the DGA cycles.
Analysis	• Involve experts in sustainability to define the research questions and parameters for systematic reviews; • Use technical experts to identify the relevant data sources; and • Rethink approaches to dietary patterns to incorporate sustainability.
Synthesis and Interpretation	• Identify topics related to sustainability so that relevant expertise during the DGSAC nomination process can be identified; and • In the report to the Secretaries, develop conclusions on the topics identified and identify research needs, evidence needs, and potential future topics related to sustainability as appropriate.
Federal Review and Update	• Incorporate conclusions into the DGA Policy Report.

NOTE: DGA = *Dietary Guidelines for Americans*; DGSAC = Dietary Guidelines Scientific Advisory Committee.
SOURCE: Presented by Barbara Schneeman on August 1, 2018; reprinted with permission.

systems approaches into the DGA. The selected strategies should then begin to be used to integrate systems mapping and modeling into the DGA process." The committee recognized that this would not "happen overnight," Schneeman said, because understanding how a systems approach can be helpful requires investment. In her opinion, a systems approach may also be a way to integrate sustainability into the DGA.

DISCUSSION

In the discussion following Schneeman's presentation, she, Springmann, Macdiarmid, Ranganathan, and Tahiri participated in an open discussion with the audience, summarized here.

Integrating Sustainability Components into the *Dietary Guidelines for Americans*

There was considerable discussion around sustainability and the DGA, beginning with Drewnowski's reminder that there are four dimensions of sustainable diets according to the FAO definition: (1) nutrition and health, (2) economic, (3) social and cultural, and (4) environmental. He expressed disappointment that the DGA have mentioned only the first of these. He stated that, to its credit, the DGAC has mentioned affordability, financial burden, and health equities in its work; however, the final documents have made no reference to these components, nor has there been any reference to societal value or food acceptance. He pointed out, for example, that among the current USDA healthy food patterns, the Mediterranean-style pattern is more expensive than the vegetarian pattern. He called for the incorporation of affordability, as well as the societal value and environmental components of sustainability, into future DGA.

In response, Schneeman reflected on the different ways in which people think about the objective of integrating sustainability into the DGA and suggested that probably everyone can bring something to the table. While acknowledging that it would be difficult with the current cycle, she encouraged the audience, "If the topics start to emerge and we have agreement on how sustainability relates to the purpose of the dietary guidelines, then we have a way to start thinking about how [to] build that into the dietary guidelines going forward."

Peter Lurie, Center for Science in the Public Interest, Washington, DC, and Food Forum member, suggested reframing Drewnowski's question in a slightly different way. Instead of asking why not, he proposed asking what is feasible. What is the likelihood that sustainability can be integrated into the DGA? Or which elements of sustainability that Drewnowski had laid out are most likely "to fall on receptive ears"? (For more detail on Drewnowski's exposition of the four dimensions of sustainability, see Chapter 2.)

Schneeman said she was unaware of which topics, other than B-24 (nutrition for children up to 24 months), will be considered in the next cycle of the DGA. She pointed to B-24 as a good case study of what it takes to bring a topic forward in a way that is suited to and positioned for the DGA process. She also commented on how the National Academies committee believed it would be helpful to move away from the practice of reviewing every topic during every DGA cycle, as there are some areas in the DGA that have not changed for 20 or 30 years (NASEM, 2017). This does not mean, she clarified, that those topics should never be reviewed, but that having a longer cycle of review for some topics would open up the opportunity to explore new topics.

Tahiri added that consumer research could help inform specific economic or social and cultural topics to include in the DGA process. In other words, it could reveal what American consumers want included in the DGA.

Rose pointed to the fact that there are two reports—the DGAC report and the final DGA. He views this as a gap given that the last DGAC report contained a chapter on sustainability that was excluded from the final DGA. He asked whether it would be possible to go back to the practice of the DGAC's issuing the final DGA without that final report being filtered through federal oversight.

Schneeman clarified that, even as far back in 1990, when she first served on the DGAC, the DGAC report went to the secretaries of HHS and USDA, who would then release the final DGA. The difference, she noted, was that the DGA at that time was a 20- or 30-page consumer pamphlet. Although its report contained a great deal of scientific detail and justification regarding any recommended DGA revisions, the DGAC was told that any new language it was recommending should be written at an eighth-grade level. Not until the 2005 DGA, Schneeman observed, was it realized that it made no sense to produce a consumer bulletin through the DGAC; rather, the DGAC's strength was conducting a scientific evaluation and examining the evidence supporting the recommendations in the DGA or any revisions thereof. Thus, she continued, it was decided that the DGAC report should serve a scientific advisory purpose and that the DGA would no longer be a consumer bulletin, but a report aimed at policy makers. It would then be the responsibility of those policy makers to develop a consumer brochure. Schneeman added that today, a federal working group reviews educational materials issued by HHS or USDA to ensure that they are consistent with the DGA. Regarding the issue of sustainability, she noted that this issue sparked a great deal of controversy in the last DGA cycle. She referred again to the report of the National Academies committee and a recommendation therein relating to the responsibility of any advisory committee that, in the process of its work, becomes aware of an issue it views as important but was not chartered to address (NASEM, 2017). Maybe that committee's job, she suggested, is to make sure that this issue is brought forward such that it will be addressed in the future, and that this, in fact, is what happened with sustainability in the last DGA. "Why are we having this discussion today?" she asked. "It is because of the controversy around how to include sustainability. Think of it as a success."

Claudia Hitja, USDA, asked whether any country had successfully integrated sustainability into its national dietary guidelines. Springmann directed Hitja to an FAO/Food Climate Research Network (FCRN) report titled *Plates, Pyramids, Planet: Developments in National Healthy and Sustainable Dietary Guidelines* (Fischer and Garnett, 2016).

Country-Level Versus Local Data

Drewnowski pointed to the correlation between the distribution of plant protein consumption across Seattle and socioeconomic status. "People who consume plant proteins are the ones who consume salad and live in nice houses on the waterfront," he observed. "When looking at grossly aggregated data by country, you really are losing track of the very small geographic distinctions." He asked Springmann how useful it is to look at country-level data.

Springmann agreed that country-level analyses examine only general trends, such as trends in what people consume or what they are thought to be eating. But that is the intent of such analyses, he asserted: to illustrate those generalities and tease out country differences, not to inform local understanding. "There are discussions to be had at any level, I suppose," he commented.

The Evidence for Successful Dietary Shifts

Curious about whether there is any evidence to suggest that sustainable diet goals will be achievable, Afshin pointed out that no country has been successful at reducing the prevalence of overweight and obesity over the past 30 years. In addition, he noted that the consumption of nuts has increased by only 2 grams over that same period. "Is it possible to increase that by 20 grams over the next 20 years?" he asked. "Has any country been able to achieve at least any of these [dietary change] scenarios over the last few years?"

At the country level, Springmann responded, this probably has not been accomplished. However, he stressed, there is evidence that specific dietary interventions can be successful. As an example, he mentioned weight loss studies conducted by Oxford University researchers demonstrating that overweight and obesity can be reduced, although success requires intensive resources and follow-up. In addition, he cited an effort in North Karelia, Finland, to reduce the intake of saturated fats, which he characterized as "pretty successful." And he suspects that there have been other, similarly successful small-scale interventions involving broad dietary changes. He also referred to an analysis of the effect of GHG taxes on food consumption. While the analysis predicted that taxing food according to its GHG emissions could influence food consumption, diets would probably not change significantly. Thus, he emphasized, "you really need a multitude of different interventions." He stressed, too, that the lack of evidence of large-scale, country-level changes does not mean there should be no efforts to achieve such changes. "I think we are called to action on all dimensions," he argued.

Tahiri suggested that by also examining socioeconomic changes, as Drewnowski had emphasized, one might in fact be able to detect country-level dietary shifts.

Ranganathan agreed with Springmann that, as she said, "there is no room for pessimism." She expressed her belief that shifts not only are possible but also can happen rapidly. She pointed to the rapid shift in people's dietary habits around meat during World War II in the United States. In the face of blockades and the need to send food to the troops, the strategy was to shift Americans at home to eating more organ meat. Ranganathan cited that as one of the most successful and rapidly implemented dietary strategies ever undertaken. Similarly, in China, she noted, there has been a campaign to reduce the use of shark fin in soup, which is traditionally seen as a food the wealthy eat. Around the globe, she added, diets are shifting in middle- and low-income countries. "We know they can shift," she said. "We just have to shift them in a more sustainable direction." She referred to the "tried and tested" private-sector strategies for shifting consumption that she had described during her presentation. "What you purchase and what ends up in your basket or on your plate is largely influenced by external forces and not necessarily what you set out to buy or eat," she observed.

In addition to the food shifts she had described earlier, Ranganathan commented on how effective marketing has shifted consumption in the area of men's grooming products as well. Her father, for example, would have considered it "not manly" to use any kind of men's grooming products other than his standard shaving equipment. But now, she pointed out, men's grooming products are a multi-billion dollar business because the companies that sell them have successfully addressed that perception. They now market the products in a manner that appeals to men's masculinity, including by packaging them, for example, in black bottles; giving them such names as "Face Fuel" and "Urban Camouflage"; and placing them on shelves next to belts or similar items. However, Ranganathan also cautioned that using only private-sector strategies is not enough; government action, policies, and price signals are also needed. But her hope is that working with businesses first, particularly food service companies, will cause them to become champions that will call for government to institute the needed changes.

Schneeman added that in the United States, the labeling of trans-fatty acids, which began in 2006, led to their elimination from packaged foods, as well as to other kinds of campaigns to remove these substances from other parts of the food sector. With respect to sugar-sweetened beverages, as far as she knows, the decline in consumption began as soon as people became aware of the need to avoid them. Both of these examples, she said, accord with Ranganathan's remarks about how changes can happen quickly. The question for her is whether these changes are occurring in a coordinated way. For example, when consumption of sugar-sweetened beverages decreased, what increased? And is the whole system responding effectively?

Springmann was asked by Rebecca Boehm, Yukon Rudd Center for Food Policy and Obesity, how interventions to reduce consumption of sugary drinks compare with interventions or approaches that might be used to reduce meat consumption. Springmann responded that this is a difficult comparison because sugary drinks are a food nobody needs, whereas meat, many people would argue, is a food that could benefit some people in low-income settings. In high-income countries, however, and also in many middle-income countries, he added, one could argue that people eat too much meat. In addition, he observed, there are many different kinds of meat. In his opinion, the difference between sugary drinks and meat does not mean that taxing meats, for example, would not work, "but it is probably not an exact parallel," he cautioned.

Tahiri emphasized the essential role of positive reinforcement. She argued that, while a range of taxes and other tools can be used, "we really should keep in mind that positive reinforcement is one thing that we should not take out of the equation of changing behaviors."

Ashley Lyles, MedPage Today, asked what role medical doctors can play in shifting behavior, specifically in getting people to change their diet. Schneeman responded that, since many consumers look to the medical profession for dietary advice, finding a way to provide advice on dietary change in that setting is important. She encouraged medical professionals to use the tools available, such as nutrition labeling; that is, help consumers in their clinics understand how to use the labeling. She pointed to dieticians as another important resource. In fact, she suggested, once a medical condition that would benefit from dietary modification has been identified, a physician might want to connect that individual with the dietitian on staff as the best resource for discussing the changes that could be made in his or her diet.

5

Innovation in Food Production and Distribution to Reduce Environmental Footprint

Session 4, moderated by Kate Houston, Cargill, Inc., Washington, DC, built on the foundation developed on the first day of the workshop while also adding some new perspectives. Speakers explored how food systems are innovating and finding new ways to address sustainability, some of which have already been implemented, Houston remarked, while others are on the horizon. This chapter summarizes the presentations and discussion that took place during this session, with highlights of the presentations provided in Box 5-1.

REDUCING THE FOOTPRINT OF ANIMAL AGRICULTURE

Frank Mitloehner, University of California, Davis, opened the session with a glimpse of what he described as "ground zero of environmental discussions, and that is the sunny state of California." He informed the audience that California is the leading agricultural state in the nation, producing 50 percent of all fruits and vegetables and 20 percent of all dairy (CDFA, 2017). What many people do not realize about California, he pointed out, is that about half of the state consists of marginal land—land that cannot be used to produce crops and is unusable for most other purposes as well, and thus is used largely for grazing livestock. Most agriculture in California occurs in the Central Valley, he noted, a place with significant environmental issues as well. He added that Fresno is not only the nation's leading agricultural county but also the one with the worst air quality (UC Agricultural Issues Center, 2009). To curb the impact not just of livestock but

BOX 5-1
Highlights of Individual Presentations*

- Improving production efficiency: implications for sustainability
  - Because the intensity of livestock production and that of greenhouse gas (GHG) emissions are inversely related, livestock production has very different environmental impacts in different parts of the world. (Mitloehner)
  - New technologies leading to improved fertility, health, genetics, and animal feeds have allowed the United States and other countries to reduce their carbon footprints through more efficient livestock production. (Mitloehner)
- Changing consumer demand: implications for sustainability
  - A shift from today's U.S. diet to what is recommended in the *Dietary Guidelines for Americans* (DGA) would have variable effects on net GHG emissions, depending on caloric intake and eating patterns (e.g., omnivore, lacto-ovo vegetarian, vegan). (Heller)
  - If one examines individual-level (National Health and Nutrition Examination Survey [NHANES] data), it is apparent that a significant reduction in GHG emissions is possible through shifts in U.S. dietary patterns. However, there are big differences between the highest and lowest emitters in terms of both calories (i.e., people whose diets contribute more to GHG emissions eat more calories) and diet composition (i.e., people whose diets contribute more to GHG emissions also eat more meat, mostly beef). (Heller)
- Restructuring food systems: implications for sustainability
  - Local and regional food systems can contribute to sustainability by strengthening economic viability, improving access to healthy foods, and creating place-based opportunities to reduce environmental burdens. (Blackstone)
  - Recycling food waste into animal feed (the "leftovers approach") can reduce GHG emissions from regional livestock systems. (Blackstone)
- The retail interface between producers and consumers: implications for sustainability
  - Food supply chains are complex, and maximizing for one outcome creates issues elsewhere. Thus, the challenges to sustainability are tremendous. Nonetheless, there are also opportunities for testing ideas and making positive changes. (Denniston)
  - From where it sits at the interface between supply chains and consumers, Walmart has learned many lessons about ways to innovate toward sustainability. (Denniston)

*These points were made by the individual workshop speakers identified above. They are not intended to reflect a consensus among workshop speakers.

of all sectors of society, California has what Mitloehner described as very aggressive regulations and among the most proactive air resources agencies.

Livestock and Climate Change: Fact or Fiction?

Mitloehner explained that, throughout his talk, he would be addressing several seemingly conflicting observations about livestock and climate change. The first is the claim that livestock is the predominant contributor of greenhouse gas (GHG) emissions globally, producing 18 percent of all anthropogenic GHG emissions, and that livestock emits more GHGs than does transportation. Mitloehner clarified that the 18 percent figure, first reported in *Livestock's Long Shadow* (FAO, 2006), was later reduced to 14.5 percent (FAO, 2013b) and that the majority of that amount is related to deforestation in developing and emerging countries. Often, he said, people will apply a global number, such as the 18 percent figure from the 2006 Food and Agriculture Organization (FAO) report, to the United States to convince others to change their eating habits. In his opinion, this is a conflating of information about global and national trends that does not hold true.

The statement that livestock emits more GHGs than does transportation also comes from the 2006 FAO report, a finding Mitloehner says he critiqued for using different methods to estimate emissions when the report was first issued. A life-cycle assessment (LCA) was used to estimate the emissions attributable to the livestock sector, taking into account all aspects of livestock production, whereas only direct emissions (i.e., from tailpipes) were used to estimate emissions from the transportation sector. Thus, Mitloehner elaborated, the LCA of the carbon footprint of a gallon of milk, for example, includes not just the direct emissions of the cow—belching or emissions from manure—but also emissions from the soil, herbicides and pesticides used to produce feed crops, the crops themselves, the feed produced from the crops, and so on. By contrast, he stated, the estimate of direct emissions for the transportation sector omitted production entirely (i.e., of cars, trucks, trains, planes, and ships), including the steel, rubber, plastic, and other materials used. Nor did it account for the construction of roads, airports, harbors, and so on. It was an "apples to oranges" comparison, Mitloehner said.

Mitloehner uses LCA in his own work. He reported that he chaired an FAO-hosted committee known as the Livestock Environmental Assessment and Performance Partnership (LEAP), which released guidelines on how to conduct LCAs for all livestock and feed commodities (FAO, 2016). Assembling these guidelines involved the work of about 300 of the world's leading LCA experts. According to Mitloehner, the guidelines are now considered the gold standard for global LCAs.

When examining GHG emissions in the United States, however, people often turn to the U.S. Environmental Protection Agency's (EPA's) inventory of direct emissions, Mitloehner continued. According to 2014 EPA data, he reported, a main contributor to the U.S. GHG inventory is carbon dioxide (CO_2) (81 percent), which he explained is a direct result mainly of fossil fuel use; other contributors include methane (11 percent), nitrous oxide (6 percent), and fluorinated gases (3 percent). Based on these data, he stated, EPA has determined that the contributors to GHG emissions in the United States are as follows: power production (i.e., electricity), 30 percent; transportation, 26 percent; industry, 21 percent; agriculture, 9 percent; commercial, 7 percent; and residential, 6 percent. He clarified that the 9 percent figure for agriculture is for all agriculture, crops and livestock combined (EPA, 2017). The U.S. livestock sector alone, which includes dairy, beef, sheep, pigs, and poultry, contributes about 4 percent to total U.S. GHG emissions. In California, that percentage is slightly higher, with the livestock sector—both beef and dairy—contributing 5.4 percent of total GHG emissions in the state (EPA, 2017). In contrast, California's transportation sector contributes 36.9 percent to the state's total GHG emissions. Mitloehner thus asserted, "The notion that livestock rivals transportation as a greenhouse gas emitter is false, particularly here in the United States."

The Largest Food-Related Contributor to Greenhouse Gases: Food Waste?

Arguably the greatest food-related contributor to GHG emissions and environmental harm overall, Mitloehner continued, is food waste. This includes not just food waste at the household level but food wasted throughout the entire food supply chain. In the United States, Mitloehner reported, 40 percent of food produced goes to waste (Gunders, 2012); globally, that figure is closer to 30 percent (FAO, 2012a).

The Growing Global Population and a Rapidly Increasing Demand for Eggs, Meat, and Milk

Mitloehner observed that the global population has been increasing exponentially since the mid-18th century and is expected to reach 10 billion by 2050. When he was a boy, there were 3.5 billion people on earth, compared with 7.6 billion today. "By the time I am an old man," he said, there will be 9.5 billion people alive. In other words, over his lifetime, the human population will have tripled. "But the natural resources to feed these people will not have tripled," he added. "If we are lucky, we will have the same amount of resources, but most likely fewer."

Today's global population growth is happening primarily in emerging and developing countries, Mitloehner continued, not only because people are having more babies but also because life expectancies are increasing, so that cumulatively, there are more people alive. He showed a satellite image of the world with much of Southeast Asia circled and stated that there are more people living inside than outside that circle. So clearly, he noted, Southeast Asia, with an expected 41 percent increase in its population over the next 10 years, is a major food security area. But, he stressed, it is not the only one: the population in Africa is expected to increase by 50 percent over the same time period, the South American population by 7 percent, and the North American population by 4 percent, while the European population is predicted to shrink slightly (Roser, 2018). "We have our work cut out for us with respect to finding means to feed a growing population without depleting our natural resources," Mitloehner said.

Mitloehner went on to point out that as the global population rises, so, too, does the demand for eggs, meat, and milk, particularly in developing parts of the world. He added that this growing demand is largely a function of disposable income, according to 2005 FAO data (see Figure 5-1), such that the higher the income, the greater the meat consumption, with the United States having the highest meat consumption per capita (kilograms [kg]/year). He predicted that, although China is on the far left of the graph in Figure 5-1, it will be at least where the United States is today in 10 years.

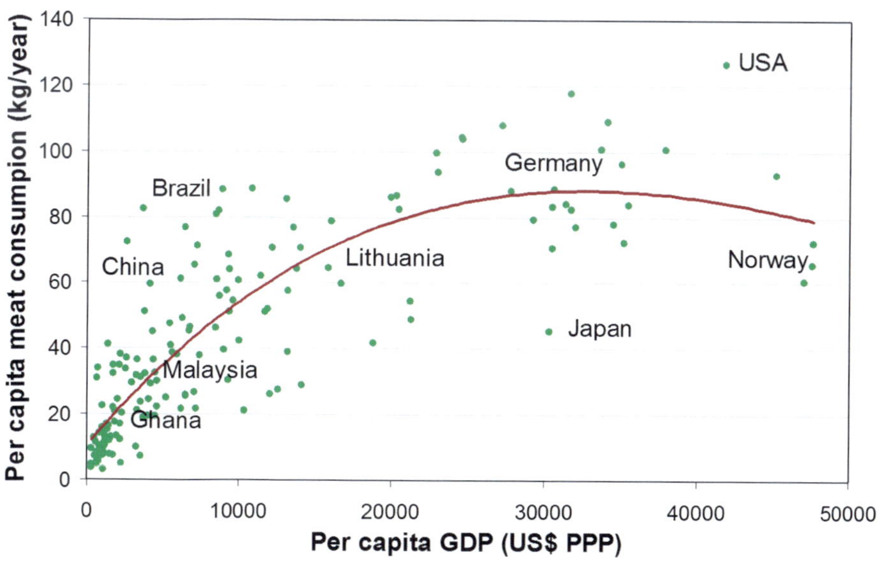

FIGURE 5-1 Meat consumption as a function of gross domestic product (GDP), by country.
NOTE: PPP = when adjusted by purchasing power parity.
SOURCES: Presented by Frank Mitloehner on August 2, 2018; FAO, 2009.

Agricultural Land Worldwide

An additional "fact or fiction?" statement that Mitloehner had cited at the beginning of his presentation was that livestock occupies 70 percent of all agricultural land globally. He clarified that while two-thirds of the world's agricultural land currently is used for livestock, particularly ruminant livestock, this is because there is no other food-producing way to use that land (FAO, 2006).

To explain, Mitloehner began by showing a map of global livestock distribution and remarked that the density of livestock in the United States (livestock units per square kilometer [km]) "pales" in comparison with that in such countries as India and China (FAO, 2006). But even more important than global livestock distribution, he continued, is the global distribution of cropland (i.e., crops grown for food for human consumption). Regardless of the number of people in the world, he stressed, whether it is 3, 7, 9, or 12 billion, "that is the only cropland we have available." To depict this problem in a different way, he asked everyone in the room to imagine that a normal (8.5 by 11 inch) piece of paper represented the surface of the Earth. He folded the paper twice, with the resulting quarter representing the total amount of land in the world. The rest, he said, is water and ice. Of that quarter-sized piece of 8.5 by 11 inch paper, he added, the equivalent of the size of a business card is the total amount of agricultural land, the rest being forests, deserts, cities, and so on. Then, he folded his business card such that one portion was two-thirds the size of the card and the other was one-third. The larger portion, he said, depicted the amount of agricultural land in the world that is considered "marginal." Again, marginal land is land that cannot be used to grow crops either because the soil is not fertile or there is not enough moisture. According to Mitloehner, the only use for that marginal land is ruminant livestock (i.e., beef, dairy, goats, sheep). Thus, only one-third of all agricultural land worldwide is so-called "arable" land, where anything can be grown (within regional limits) (Alexandratos and Bruinsma, 2012).

To further illustrate the importance of the livestock sector with respect to the global food supply, Mitloehner added that not only is most agricultural land not arable, but half of all arable land in the world is fertilized with chemical fertilizers and the other half with organic fertilizers, which are, by and large, animal manure (FAO, 2006).

The Inverse Relationship Between Production Intensity and Intensity of Greenhouse Gas Emissions

A final "fact or fiction?" statement cited by Mitloehner at the beginning of his talk was that grazing systems produce fewer GHG emissions relative to conventional animal production in confinement systems. He explained that cows that produce very little milk have a very large carbon footprint relative to those that produce large amounts of milk (see Figure 5-2). He added that this is because the amount of nutrients fed to a cow that produces very little milk (on the left side of the graph in Figure 5-2) is used largely to keep her alive (i.e., "maintenance requirements"), whereas the carbon footprint of a cow that produces a large amount of milk (on the right side of the graph in Figure 5-2) is "diluted" through the amount of milk she produces.

In the United States, Mitloehner continued, about 25,000 pounds of milk is produced per cow per year, while in India and Mexico, respectively, it takes about 20 and about 5 cows to produce the same amount of milk (FAO, 2017a). He emphasized the vast differences in the cumulative environmental impact of 1 versus 5 versus 20 cows, highlighting FAO data from 2010 showing that North America is not the highest, as many think, but the lowest of any region of the world with respect to GHG emissions per unit of milk produced. He remarked that if U.S. data were to be teased out of that combined North American dataset, the difference between milk production emissions in the United States and elsewhere in the world would be starker. The same is true, he observed, with respect to emission intensities associated

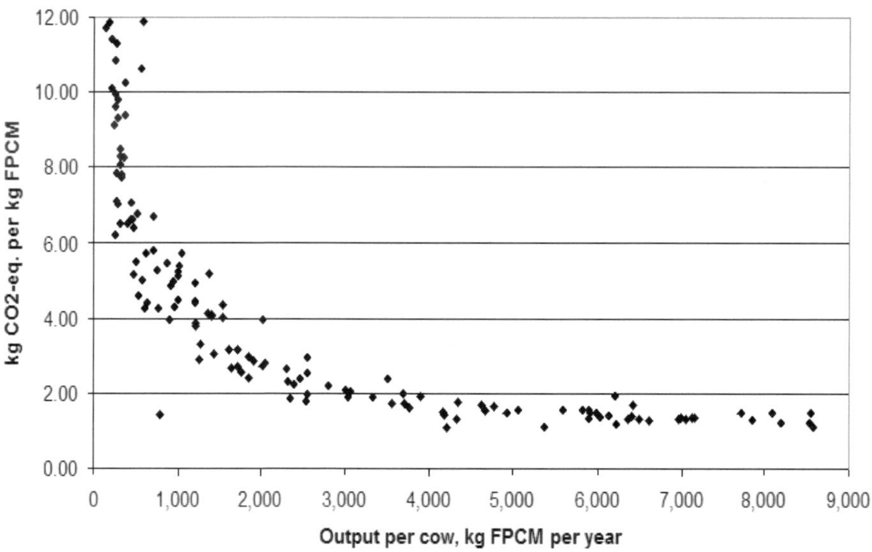

FIGURE 5-2 Greenhouse gas emissions (kilograms [kg] of carbon dioxide [CO_2]-equivalent) per kg fat- and protein-corrected milk (FPCM) as a function of output per cow (kg FPCM per year).
SOURCES: Presented by Frank Mitloehner on August 2, 2018, modified from Gerber et al., 2011.

with both ruminant and nonruminant animals used for meat, with U.S. totals being lower than those in Brazil, China, the European Union, and India.

The Important Role of Technology

According to Mitloehner, the fact that the United States has the lowest, not highest, carbon footprint in the world with respect to beef, dairy, and nonruminant meat animals per unit of product is a function of four approaches: (1) reproductive efficiency; (2) improved health, including vaccination and treatment of animals; (3) improved genetics, meaning that what he termed "high-merit" genetics are being applied to both animals and plants; and (4) the feeding of more energy-dense diets to animals (Gill et al., 2010).

"These four tools have allowed us to shrink animal herds to historic levels in this country," Mitloehner continued. In 1950, he observed, there were 25 million dairy cows across the United States, whereas today there are 9 million. Yet, even with fewer cows, he explained, the United States is producing 60 percent more milk with this much smaller herd; thus, the carbon footprint of a glass of milk is two-thirds smaller today than it was 70 years ago. The same is true of beef, he added: in 1970, there were 140 million head of beef in the United States; today there are 90 million, so 50 million fewer, yet the same amount of beef is produced as in 1970 (i.e., 24 million tons). The same is true yet again of pork, he observed, with pork production in the United States having tripled over the past 60 years (Mitloehner, 2016). "This is a vast improvement in performance," he said, leading to significant reductions in environmental emissions.

Other Animals (Outside of Agriculture), Other Countries

Mitloehner commented on the 9.5 million horses in the United States, compared with the country's 9 million dairy cows, and the lack of discussion around their environmental footprint. Nor does anyone talk about the 160 million dogs and cats nationwide, he added, which consume the same amount of food as 70 million people (Okin, 2007). Mitloehner clarified that he did not mean to deflect from livestock's contribution by making these statements, but simply wanted to provide additional perspective.

Also to provide additional perspective, Mitloehner described the current situation with swine in China, home to half the world's pig population and a staggering 1 billion pigs produced per year (Wang, 2006). For Mitloehner, even more remarkable than the number of pigs produced annually is their preweaning mortality. Each year, 40 percent of China's pig crop, or 400 million pigs, die preweaning and never make it to market. According to Mitloehner, the situation is even worse in India and in African countries because the veterinary systems are dysfunctional, genetics are poor, and the animals' nutrition is insufficient. He noted that the Intergovernmental Panel on Climate Change (IPCC) has estimated that about 70 to 80 percent of the global emissions impact of livestock occurs in developing countries because of production inefficiencies (Lubungu, 2017).

Final Remarks

In summary, Mitloehner highlighted two key points. First, livestock has very different environmental footprints throughout the world, with technologies having allowed the United States and other countries with efficient livestock production to arrive at where they are today. The state of California, for example, has mandated a 40 percent reduction in GHG emissions in the next 12 years. "It will be achieved," Mitloehner asserted. He mentioned technologies being developed to reduce enteric emissions from animals, which constitute the major agricultural source of methane, and technologies being used to digest manure anaerobically so as to convert it into power and fuel. Second, he pointed to the inverse relationship between production intensity and emission intensity, such that the more efficient the agricultural production, the smaller is the environmental footprint. The same is true of vehicles, he observed: the more fuel-efficient a vehicle is, the less gas it burns and the fewer emissions it releases.

REDUCING THE FOOTPRINT THROUGH ALTERNATIVE DIETS

Martin Heller, University of Michigan, Ann Arbor, revisited some of what had been discussed on the first day of the workshop about the impact of diet on the environment, but with a focus on U.S., not global, trends. He described several different approaches that have been used to predict how potential shifts in the U.S. diet could reduce the environmental impacts of the food system.

Why Consider Diets?

Heller's starting point for thinking about the role of diet was a collection of studies comparing projections of population growth and food demand with what predictive models indicate is needed to reduce global GHG emissions and avoid dangerous climate change. According to Heller, these studies have shown repeatedly that production-side improvements will be insufficient to meet the target of a 2°C rise in global temperature (Bajželj et al., 2014; Bennetzen et al., 2016; Bryngelsson et al., 2016; Hedenus et al., 2014). For example, Hedenus and colleagues (2014) predict that by 2050–2070, food requirements for the world's growing population will occupy most of the available GHG emissions space if the world is to remain within the 2°C "safe zone." But that same space, Heller stressed, requires room for other sectors as well (energy, transportation, industry, land use changes). He noted that adding increased agricultural productivity to the model, such as what Mitloehner had discussed, or technical mitigation measures, such as manure management, would reduce the portion of the available emissions space occupied by agricultural emissions, but there still would not be enough room for the other sectors. He interpreted these findings to mean that demand-side reductions are also necessary if the world is to stay within that 2°C safe zone. By demand-side reductions, he meant reduced animal-based food, specifically reduced meat and dairy consumption, and reduced food waste. As previous speakers had, he pointed to the large differences in GHG emissions between plant-based and animal-based foods. Heller noted that, while it may not always be appropriate to compare GHG emissions per weight (kilogram), doing so provides at least a scale for comparison (see Chapter 2 for a summary of Drewnowski's remarks on comparing GHG emissions by weight versus calories).

What Would Happen If the United States Shifted to the Diet Recommended by the *Dietary Guidelines for Americans*?

Heller next considered what would happen if the U.S. diet shifted to that recommended by the *Dietary Guidelines for Americans* (DGA). He described how he and a colleague compared the 2010 U.S. diet, based on the U.S. Department of Agriculture's (USDA's) Loss-Adjusted Food Availability dataset as a proxy, with an average per capita intake of 2,534 calories, against the 2010 DGA food patterns for both 2,534 calories and 2,000 calories (which is closer to what is recommended) (Heller and Keoleian, 2014a). He noted, first, that while the estimated 2010 per capita caloric intake may seem excessive, it was what the data revealed; and second, that although the 2010 DGA is now outdated, the changes between it and the 2015 DGA were subtle and likely would not influence the results.

The researchers found that with the current U.S. diet, GHG emissions associated with meat (beef, pork, and lamb) make up 48 percent of total diet-related GHG emissions. Beef accounts for 84 percent of that figure, so 40 percent of total diet-related GHG emissions is attributable to beef. Heller explained further that dairy contributes 20 percent of total diet-related GHG emissions, while plant-based foods contribute another 22 percent. He added that if the American diet shifted toward what is recommended, which would include increases in consumption of fruits and vegetables, seafood, and dairy (for the omnivorous DGA pattern), there would be a notable decrease in emissions associated with meat, poultry, and eggs, but also a notable increase in emissions related to dairy and slight increases in emissions attributable to fruit and vegetable consumption. The net effect, Heller stated, would be a 12 percent increase in GHG emissions for a 2,534-calorie diet and a 1 percent decrease for a 2,000-calorie diet (Heller and Keoleian, 2014a).

Heller and Keoleian (2014a) carried their analyses through to the lacto-ovo vegetarian and vegan DGA patterns, as well as Harvard's Healthy Eating Plate (see Table 5-1). Heller explained that the latter is similar to the omnivorous DGA pattern, but with less red meat and dairy.[1] For a 2,000-calorie diet, the researchers found that, compared with an omnivorous diet, with its 1 percent decrease in GHG emissions, a shift to a vegan diet or to either a lacto-ovo vegetarian or Harvard's Healthy Eating Plate diet would reduce GHG emissions by 53 percent and 33 percent, respectively, compared with the current average American diet.

What Heller found interesting about the latter findings is that the reduction associated with Harvard's Healthy Eating Plate, which still contains meat, is the same as that associated with the lacto-ovo vegetarian diet, which contains no meat. Thus, he said, "we don't need to necessarily think about all or nothing—vegetarian or bust."

GHG Impacts of Food Waste

"Of course," Heller continued, "everything I've showed you so far looks at just the consumed portion of the food" people eat. He noted that

TABLE 5-1 Comparison of Greenhouse Gas (GHG) Emissions from the Current U.S. Diet Versus Various Recommended Diets, at Intake of 2,000 Calories per Day

Eating Pattern	GHG Emissions (kg CO_2 equivalent/capita per day)	Reduction from Current "Average" Diet (%)
2010 DGA omnivorous	3.6	1
2010 DGA lacto-ovo vegetarian	2.4	33
2010 DGA vegan	1.7	53
Harvard's Healthy Eating Plate	2.4	33

NOTE: CO_2 = carbon dioxide; DGA = *Dietary Guidelines for Americans*; kg = kilogram.
SOURCES: Presented by Martin Heller on August 2, 2018, modified from Heller and Keoleian, 2014a.

[1]The Healthy Eating Plate "is characterized by high quality grains (whole vs. refined), healthy proteins (fish, poultry, beans and nuts vs. red meat and processed meat), greater intake of poly unsaturated fatty acids (healthy oils), reduced intake of sugar-sweetened beverages, and reduced dairy" (Heller and Keoleian, 2014b).

one-third of total U.S. diet-related emissions are from food waste (Heller and Keoleian, 2014a), an amount equivalent to the tailpipe emissions from 33 million average passenger vehicles.

Heller explained that this one-third estimate does not include GHG emissions associated with disposing of food waste, only those associated with producing the wasted food. If one accounts for disposal and assumes that all food waste is disposed of in landfills, which he recognizes is not true but cited for perspective, the estimate of GHG emissions attributable to food waste would increase by another 30 percent (Heller and Keoleian, 2014a).

Other Studies and Approaches to Examining the Environmental Impact of Dietary Shifts

Heller went on to observe that other studies have taken a similar approach to using food availability data to compare GHG emissions associated with the current diet against recommended diets. As just one example, he cited the work of Tom and colleagues (2016), who considered two additional environmental impact indicators—water use and energy use—in addition to GHG emissions. They found that a shift to a recommended food mix would increase GHG emissions by 6 percent, energy use by 28 percent, and water use by 10 percent.

Heller then described the work of Peters and colleagues (2016), who, instead of looking at GHG emissions, examined the carrying capacity of U.S. agricultural land (i.e., the number of persons that can be fed from an area of land). Like Heller and Keoleian (2014a), they estimated current consumption using the USDA Loss-Adjusted Food Availability dataset as their baseline. They then combined average crop yields and livestock rations to determine how much land is required to feed the U.S. population both currently and under a range of different recommended diets. According to Heller, they found that the current carrying capacity of U.S. agricultural land is about 130 percent of the 2010 population. If the American diet shifted to the DGA-recommended omnivorous diet, that figure would increase to 136 percent of the 2010 population; if the diet shifted to 80 percent omnivorous and 20 percent lacto-ovo vegetarian, which Heller described as "a little better than Meatless Monday," the figure would increase to 178 percent; if the diet shifted to 20 percent omnivorous and 80 percent lacto-ovo vegetarian, it would increase to 249 percent; and if all animal products were eliminated, so that the diet shifted to 100 percent vegan, it would increase to 238 percent (Peters et al., 2016). In other words, Heller clarified, eliminating *all* animal agriculture would mean less carrying capacity than having some animal agriculture. However, he pointed out, significant reductions in animal-based foods in the U.S. diet would be necessary before one would begin to see the positive effects of utilizing marginal lands through animal agriculture.

Individual-Level Analysis

"But all of that is looking at the U.S. diet as an average," Heller continued. Analyzing diet at the individual level, he stated, "opens up a lot of possibilities." One can begin linking diet, health, and environmental impacts across a population and, he pointed out, "really set the stage for some more nuanced modeling of dietary change." He went on to describe his recent work linking GHG emissions and energy use to individual self-selected diets.

Using 2005–2010 National Health and Nutrition Examination Survey (NHANES) data for 16,800 individuals, Heller and colleagues (2018) linked more than 7,000 as-consumed food items to their environmental impacts. They conducted an exhaustive search of the LCA literature to populate a database they called dataFIELD (database of Food Impacts on the Environment for Linking to Diets). Because most of the available LCA literature is based on food commodities, Heller and his team also relied on a Food Commodities Intake Database to represent the 7,000 as-consumed food items as compositions of roughly 300 food commodities. Finally, they linked data in dataFIELD with NHANES data to estimate diet-related GHG emissions per capita, including the contribution of both consumed food and food loss (both retail and consumer losses, using data from additional sources). They examined energy use associated with food production in a similar way.

At the mean of the population, Heller reported, total GHG emissions were 4.7 kg CO_2-equivalent per capita per day (3.6 kg CO_2-equivalent per capita per day for consumed food; 0.3 kg CO_2-equivalent per capita per day for retail losses; 0.9 kg CO_2-equivalent per capita per day for consumer losses) and 2.2 kg CO_2-equivalent per capita per 1,000 kilocalories (kcal) (1.7 kg CO_2-equivalent per capita per 1,000 kcal for consumed food; 0.1 kg CO_2-equivalent per capita per 1,000 kcal for retail losses; 0.4 kg CO_2-equivalent per capita per 1,000 kcal for consumer losses).

But again in Heller's opinion, the really interesting conclusions from this work derive from being able to look at GHG emissions as a distribution across a population (see Figure 5-3). He and his research team found that when individual diets are ranked by GHG emissions and the population is divided into quintiles based on those rankings (with bottom emitters in the 1st quintile and top emitters in the 5th quintile), there is an eight-fold difference in cumulative emissions between the top and bottom emitters (see Figure 5-4). For Heller, that difference is striking. "We knew there

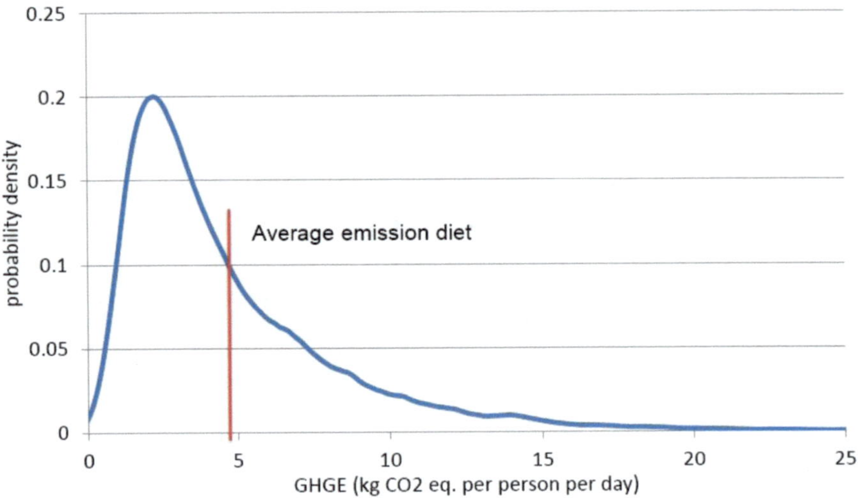

FIGURE 5-3 Distribution of greenhouse gas emissions (GHGEs) from production of nationally representative 1-day diets.
SOURCES: Presented by Martin Heller on August 2, 2018, modified from Heller et al., 2018.

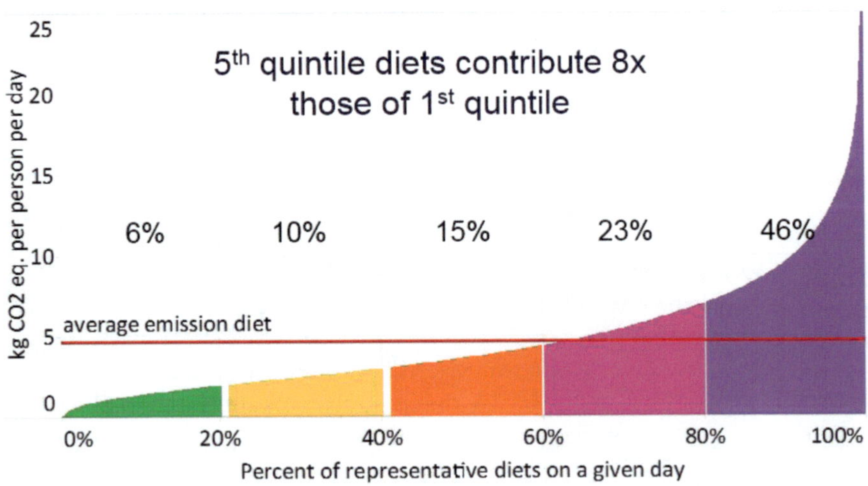

FIGURE 5-4 Cumulative greenhouse gas emission intensity of U.S. 1-day diets, divided into quintiles.
SOURCES: Presented by Martin Heller on August 2, 2018, modified from Heller et al., 2018.

was going to be variance," he said, "but it is much greater than we were anticipating."

What is driving those differences? First, according to Heller, are notable differences in total caloric intake, with top emitters eating more calories (see Figure 5-5). But even when caloric intake is normalized, he observed, there remains a five-fold difference in GHG emissions between the top and bottom emitters, which suggests a difference in diet composition as well. In fact, as shown in Figure 5-5, a much greater percentage of GHG emissions from top emitters is attributable to meat (70 percent) relative to bottom emitters (27.1 percent). The majority of meat-associated emissions by top emitters is attributable to beef (64 percent of total emissions), compared with poultry for the bottom emitters (15 percent of total emissions) (Heller et al., 2018).

Heller described average beef consumption as 51 grams per day—roughly the equivalent of eating a quarter pounder every other day. In contrast, individuals in the top quintile (the top emitters) consume about one-third of a pound of beef daily. If those in the upper quintile were to shift their diet to one associated with average emissions through some combination of diet composition and caloric intake reduction, Heller suggested, the environmental savings in terms of GHG emissions after 1 year would be equivalent to 44.6 million Americans driving 15 miles fewer every day, a

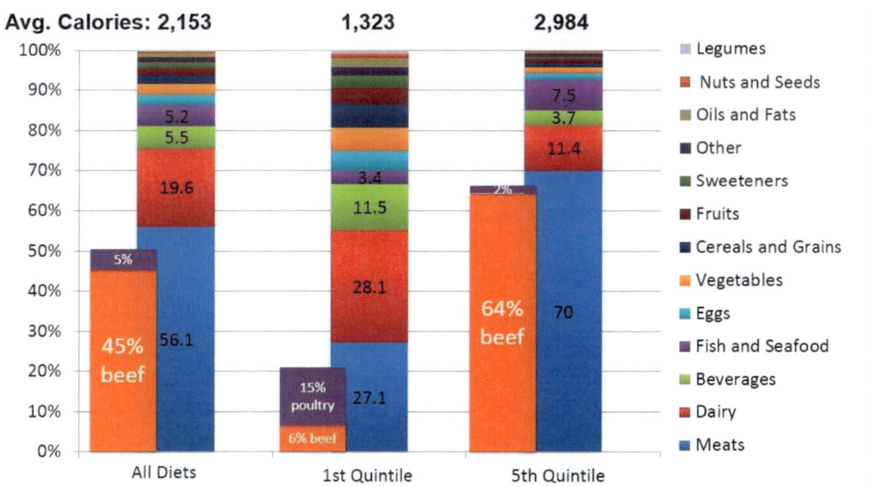

FIGURE 5-5 Percentage contributions from food groups to total greenhouse gas emissions for all diets, 1st-quintile diets (bottom emitters), and 5th-quintile diets (top emitters).
SOURCES: Presented by Martin Heller on August 2, 2018, modified from Heller et al., 2018.

reduction that could bring the United States 10 percent closer to achieving the United Nations (UN) climate targets (Heller et al., 2018).

Final Remarks

In conclusion, Heller highlighted several key points. First, demand-side changes likely are needed to meet emission-reduction targets, even with some of the efficiency improvements and technological advances discussed by Mitloehner. Second, the individual-level modeling he had described points to wide discrepancies in the United States with respect to the diet-related impact on GHG emissions and offers a different lens for thinking about policy scenarios. Finally, Heller acknowledged having provided a one-sided look at environmental impacts—namely, a look at GHG emissions. He emphasized that there are other environmental indicators, such as water and land use, as well as other aspects of sustainability, that need to be considered.

LOCAL AND REGIONAL FOOD SYSTEMS IN SUSTAINABLE DIETS

Nicole Tichenor Blackstone, Tufts University, Boston, Massachusetts, reflected on the difference between research on sustainable diets and research on local and regional food systems, and how this difference underlies the reality that there are multiple ways to think about sustainable food systems. As an example of her work in research on sustainable diets, she mentioned an analysis in which she and her colleagues compared the environmental impacts of three different diet patterns in the most recent DGA (Blackstone et al., 2018). She pointed out that this kind of analysis is different from the type of work that researchers who study local and regional food systems, including she herself, often do. Yet, she observed that both types of research serve as approaches to understanding sustainable diets, an idea that she traced to Garnett (2014).

Garnett (2014) identifies three different perspectives, or lenses, through which researchers think about sustainable food systems: demand restraint, efficiency-oriented, and food systems transformation. Blackstone explained that demand restraint had also been discussed by several previous speakers—that is, how diets can be shifted or how consumer behavior can be influenced to reduce the environmental, social, and economic costs of the food that is produced and consumed. She identified the second perspective, efficiency-oriented, as what Mitloehner had been getting at—that is, how technology and innovation can be used to reduce the environmental, social, and economic impacts of agriculture and related supply chains. She then turned to the third perspective, which Garnett (2014) terms food systems transformation. The central argument of this perspective, she explained, is that the problems, or externalities, of the food system are the result of the social and economic organization of the system, rather than being just technical problems or the result of individual decisions.

Blackstone announced that the remainder of her talk would focus on the third perspective—food systems transformation—and expressed the hope that bringing this perspective to the workshop would result in the continuation of conversation around it. Specifically, she said she would focus on local and regional food systems and their economic, social, human health, and environmental contributions to sustainability. People who work in local and regional food systems consider themselves food systems transformers, she said, because they are exploring alternative ways to organize farms and supply chains.

What Is a Local Food System?

According to Blackstone, there is no single definition of a local or regional food system, but one element that runs through all the different definitions is geography. In some cases, she elaborated, this element is distance; in other cases, it is a mileage radius; and in still other cases, it is state-based. Sometimes, she observed, these systems are defined around marketing channels. Indeed, she noted, this is how USDA tracks local and regional food systems: food being sold through either direct or intermediated marketing channels. She explained that direct-to-consumer marketing includes farms selling directly to consumers in farmers' markets, at farm stands, or through community-supported agricultural endeavors, while intermediated marketing includes farms selling to institutions, retailers, or regional distributors ("hubs"). She identified perceived attributes as yet another way of defining local and regional food systems (Johnson et al., 2013). She emphasized the word "perceived," noting that many people who are highly enthusiastic about local food sometimes incorporate perceived attributes into their definition of local or regional systems regardless of whether those attributes are valid. For example, they may perceive local foods as having better quality or safety; as automatically being sourced from small-scale farms; or as being fairer, more just, or better for the environment.

Local Versus Regional

With respect to the difference between local and regional, Blackstone remarked that the regional level encompasses the local level, and is typically larger and more comprehensive (Clancy and Ruhf, 2010). She explained that she works on regional food systems in the northeastern United States that cover 12 states, extending from Maine to West Virginia.

Local Food Systems in the United States

Blackstone observed that local and regional food systems represent a very small fraction of the overall U.S. food system—only about 8 percent of U.S. farms use direct or intermediated marketing channels, totaling about $6.1 billion (2012), a little less than 2 percent of U.S. agricultural sales (Low et al., 2015). She added that most local and regional foods are sold through intermediated channels, as opposed to direct markets, and that about half of all local and regional foods are produce, while 30 percent are animal products.

How Might Local and Regional Food Systems Contribute to Sustainability?

Blackstone discussed three ways in which local and regional food systems might contribute to sustainability: (1) economic viability, (2) access and health, and (3) the environment. She went on to discuss each of these in detail, but focused mainly on environmental implications.

Economic Viability

According to Blackstone, research has shown that farms working in local supply chains can have higher net revenue relative to those working in mainstream chains (King et al., 2010). Research has also shown that farms using direct marketing channels have higher survival rates compared with those using intermediate channels (Low et al., 2015). Regarding the latter finding, Blackstone explained that farms with higher survival rates are those with positive sales over time, a notable fact given that U.S. farms have a fairly low rate of positive sales over time. Also notable, she suggested, is that Low and colleagues (2015) found this association to obtain across scale, from very small to midscale to large farms, and for beginning farmers as well. She stressed that beginning farmers in particular are critical for sustainability in agriculture given the aging farmer population. "We need to keep folks on the land," she declared. In her opinion, these findings are promising for creating future opportunities for farmers.

Blackstone identified food hubs as another opportunity for small and midscale producers who are often locked out of mainstream (i.e., large-scale retail and global) markets because they struggle to meet quantity, quality, or consistency requirements. She defined food hubs, of which there are more than 300 in the United States, as entities that aggregate, market, and distribute source-identified food and often have a values-based mission to support small and midscale farms. She referred to the *2017 National Food Hub Report* as a source of information on these entities and their contribution to the economic viability of these small and midscale operations (Colasanti et al., 2018).

Access and Health

Regarding access to healthier, plant-based foods, Blackstone remarked that there is some evidence at the national level indicating that prices for selected produce items, such as tomatoes, potatoes, and some other fruits and vegetables, may be lower at farmers' markets than at retail outlets, including superstores (Low et al., 2015). She clarified, however, that these lower prices are only one dimension of access. Shopping at farmers' markets requires a dedicated trip, time, and motivation. "So it's not an end-all, be-all for access," she said, but "there may be some price benefits."

In addition, Blackstone reported, emerging evidences suggests that local food interventions, such as farm-to-school programs and other similarly complex interventions (i.e., programs that combine multiple factors, such as gardens, nutrition education, taste tests, and food variety) can result in modest increases in fruit and vegetable consumption, as well as increased willingness to try and increased liking of different fruits and vegetables (Graziose and Ang, 2018; Izumi et al., 2015).

Environment: Transportation

In some cases, Blackstone observed, the transportation footprint of a food is greater when the supply chain is local (Low et al., 2015; Nicholson et al., 2015). The reason is that local supply chains can have lower fuel efficiency per unit product; because of their larger scale, regional food systems may offer efficiency advantages (King et al., 2010).

Blackstone emphasized, however, that transportation in food miles is only a small part of the overall environmental footprint of foods. With some exceptions (e.g., air freight for some commodities), she reported, food miles contribute only about 5 percent of average weekly household food-related GHG emissions. Most household food-related GHG emissions, she elaborated, are centered around the farming and manufacturing of foods (Boehm et al., 2018).

Environment: Beef Production in the Northeast

In the northeastern United States, Blackstone continued, not only is there a great deal of interest in local meat, but the region also has a culturally and economically significant dairy sector. She explained that the dairy sector is a multifunctional system that produces both milk and beef, and that the beef it produces has a lower overall environmental footprint compared with regional grass-fed beef production and uses less land than conventional beef production (Tichenor et al., 2017). "So there are ways in which regionally specific production systems might have some environmental benefits," she said, "depending on where you are in the region."

Yet, Blackstone pointed out, these systems rely heavily on corn-based feeds. She and her research team were struck by evidence in the animal science literature demonstrating that a high-energy feed that mimics corn can be created from plant-based retail food waste (Froetschel et al., 2014), coupled with the large potential supply of plant-based retail food waste in the Northeast because of the large number of urban centers. They therefore wondered whether there might be a way to further improve the sustainability of these systems by using food waste as feed. Currently, Blackstone noted, policies to promote green energy or less landfilling of waste in the region are encouraging anaerobic digestion of food waste, and that policy pressure is growing. But again, she asked, what if, instead of sending that food waste to the digesters, it were used in animal feed? Would there be net benefits? So she and her team conducted an LCA of the benefits and costs of shifting food waste to feed and found that doing so would indeed reduce both GHG emissions and acidification potential (Blackstone et al., in prep).

Blackstone referred to this as a "leftovers approach" because it relies both on leftovers from the dairy industry to produce beef and leftovers from human consumption and retail for animal feed. In her opinion, the recycling of food waste into feed should be a priority across the region. She called for further assessment of the feasibility of using this leftovers approach with additional species, such as pigs.

Environment: System-Level Issues

"As we think about folks shifting to more sustainable diets," Blackstone cautioned, "we need to think about where that's going to happen." She explained that production of fruits and vegetables in the United States is highly geographically concentrated, as Mitloehner had pointed out. She noted that California produces most of the country's leafy greens (95 percent from Arizona and California combined), broccoli (92 percent), celery (95 percent), garlic (100 percent), processing tomatoes (94 percent), strawberries (79 percent), and grapes (89 percent) (CDFA, 2017). And because fruits and vegetables are major contributors to consumptive water use and water depletion (Blackstone et al., 2018), increasing fruit and vegetable production in current production centers such as California would exacerbate water stress in those areas. She added that, because geographically concentrated production is increasingly vulnerable to climate change–related droughts, fires, and erratic weather patterns, concentrated production centers are likely to be less resilient in the face of these shocks. She suggested thinking about how local and regional food systems might be potential mechanisms for increasing fruit and vegetable production in sustainable ways, though she acknowledged that this was only a hypothesis and that much empirical work would be needed to understand its implications.

Questions to Consider

Blackstone listed several questions to consider as research in the field of sustainable diets moves forward. First, how can the potential contributions of local and regional food systems be integrated into such research in meaningful ways? Blackstone suggested involving sociologists to help examine the social and cultural potential of these alternative systems. Second, what is the role of circular economies (e.g., using food waste as feed)? Going beyond the food system, how does that system intersect with other aspects of the economy, and how can more circular systems be created? Third, Blackstone urged consideration of how decentralizing production might contribute to resilience, something she believes should be studied empirically. Finally, she asked about structural issues and the underlying economic and social systems driving the externalities that exist today.

In conclusion, Blackstone stressed that local and regional food systems are not the answer to all sustainability issues. In her opinion, achieving sustainable diets will require many different approaches and all scales working together—from global and large-volume distributors, to farmers' markets, to backyard gardens.

SUSTAINABLE FOOD SYSTEMS: INNOVATIONS AT THE INTERSECTION OF SUPPLY CHAINS AND CONSUMERS

For Karrie Denniston, Walmart, Bentonville, Arkansas, there are any number of different doors one could walk through when thinking about the role retail serves in sustainable food systems. "Should we talk about food waste? Should we talk about global policy? Should we talk about local systems?" she asked. Regardless of which door one walks through, she suggested, the issues very quickly become muddled, and "you will very quickly run into someone else walking through a different door." The consequences of this complexity, she asserted, are that "when we maximize for one thing, we create issues somewhere else." For example, as Blackstone had pointed out, increasing fruit and vegetable consumption creates issues of water stress. As another example, packaging food differently to extend shelf life creates plastic waste. Denniston informed the audience that the focus of her presentation would be how retail sits at a nexus amid all of these different issues, and on where Walmart enters into the conversation.

Walmart's Mission and the Creation of Shared Value

According to Denniston, Walmart has about 11,000 stores around the globe, plus multiple e-commerce platforms. The company serves about 27 countries and 270 million customers yearly, and it sources from about 100 different countries worldwide. "So that's an unbelievably complex system," Denniston said. "We end up being this interface between supply chain and demand, because we see the customer as they walk through the door and we play this signaling role, sending [signals] back and forth between where supply chains are at and where customers are going."

With respect to Walmart's mission "to save people money so that they can live better," Denniston reflected on the fact that while some markers of global prosperity are moving in positive directions, inequality is increasing. And as consumption demand continues to increase, so will the pressure around affordability and access as more people want more things. "Price will continue to matter," Denniston observed. She added that the growing global population is expected to exacerbate the already large impact of consumption on the environment and will raise new social issues as well.

In terms of where Walmart fits into this picture for the long term, Denniston stated that it sees itself as creating shared value. "By that," she said, "we think that doing good in the world is actually also good for business," and without surety of supply, resources, and sustainable food systems, there would be no business. Thus, Walmart's aspiration is to bring safe, healthy, affordable food to people in places where they need it through cold chain,[2] logistic support, and other improvements and in a way that is regenerative to the environment and is good for both the people who eat and the people who produce the food. Denniston stressed, however, that no one business or any one sector, academic or nongovernmental organization (NGO), can do this alone; changes in infrastructure, as well as in behavior, will be required. She added that Walmart cannot focus on everything everywhere because it sources from so many countries worldwide and from so many different types of supply chains. Therefore, it prioritizes its contribution to these efforts based on where the greatest risk lies (i.e., the potential for things to go wrong), the tools at its disposal (e.g., suppliers, logistics expertise), its philanthropic tools (e.g., where it can fill a gap or scale a promising program that does not yet have market viability or government support to scale on its own), and customer feedback.

[2]The term "cold chain" refers to a temperature-controlled supply chain. For more information, see https://www.who.int/countries/eth/areas/immunization/epi_logistics/en/index1.html (accessed January 4, 2019).

The Complexity of Supply Chains

Denniston cited seafood as a good example of how the social and environmental implications of supply chains are so inextricably linked. Think about shrimp, she suggested. Shrimp grown in aquaculture ponds need to be fed protein. That protein comes from what is known in the industry as "trash fish"—food that is fished out of the sea and lands on a boat, but has no market value because it is not a species people like to buy. It is on those boats far back in the supply chain where that fishmeal is being caught that the greatest risk of exploitation exists for workers—for example, having their passports withheld and being forced to work long hours. Denniston emphasized the relative lack of visibility that far back in the supply chain. "That's a key issue as we think about sustainable food systems," she stressed, "what's happening to those folks on those boats." But then shift the lens, she said, to the person who is captaining that boat. That captain is going to fish for a longer period of time just to get the same catch that meets his economic needs.

On another boat farther up the supply chain, Denniston continued, fishing for some other species, a crew is trying to meet all the standards of sustainable certification. She described them as really wanting to "do it the right way." So they pull up their catch and take it to port, but then the wholesaler to whom they bring it does not have enough demand to keep it separated from other catches, and their catch never makes it to market with a signal saying, "we worked hard to catch this sustainably."

Meanwhile, in a nearby village, Denniston said, imagine a farmer who has worked hard to perfect what she has been doing with her aquaculture ponds. Yet, her neighbor has not been judicious about water quality or pond runoff. Consequently, her ponds become diseased, and her harvest fails.

Denniston then pointed to a family somewhere around the world that walks into a store and sees information about what seafood can provide them in terms of health, but they are worried that they are unable to afford it. The challenge, she said, is not only how to communicate healthy food messages so that people can navigate the information, but also how to provide access to that healthy food. She noted that it is because of this challenge that Walmart and the Walmart Foundation made a commitment to help provide 4 billion meals over 5 years to people in need.

In summarizing her supply chain example, Denniston said, "We took a trip around the world, and all of those individuals, all of those communities, are acting completely rationally ... doing what they are doing." Yet, she stressed, the challenges they face are tremendous. At the same time, however, so, too, are the opportunities. "We can walk through any of these doors and test ideas, test tools, test innovations, and create positive changes," Denniston observed. For the remainder of her presentation, she discussed some of the lessons Walmart has learned when entering these doors and encountering these issues.

Lessons Learned by Working Across Supply Chains

Denniston described six lessons learned by working across supply chains: (1) what good looks like must be defined, (2) industry collaboration is necessary to strengthen market systems, (3) transparency and data matter, (4) engage the people who are impacted by the issues, (5) economics help drive innovation, and (6) consumer engagement helps drive demand.

What Good Looks Like Must Be Defined

In Denniston's opinion, defining what good looks like is a powerful tool as it points people in the same direction toward what should be done. Dietary guidelines are an example, as is the Paris Agreement's 2°C goal. An example from the Walmart Foundation is its investment in small and medium enterprises in China to help them understand how to mitigate food safety risks. The first step toward doing that, Denniston observed, was helping them understand food safety practices: only after a shared understanding and food safety code were agreed upon could training begin.

Industry Collaboration Is Necessary to Strengthen Market Systems

A second lesson learned, Denniston continued, is the importance of bringing people together to drive change. She cited as an example Walmart's work on what is called the Midwest Road Collaborative, whereby suppliers; local community leaders; and others across Illinois, Iowa, and Nebraska come together to decide collectively how to optimize fertilizer, reduce nutrient runoff, and improve water quality. She suggested that if Walmart had simply approached those same suppliers and requested that they implement sustainable practices, it would have meant nothing to them. The market signal is not strong enough for one farmer to act alone, she stressed. Rather, "it's the collaboration that makes the difference."

Transparency and Data Matter

"What we measure matters," Denniston continued, since the greater is the visibility into a supply chain, the greater is the opportunity to respond. She relayed how in 2017, Walmart started piloting block chain technology as a tool for understanding food systems more rapidly. But before initiating the pilot, her staff asked a team to identify where a specific package of mangoes had originated—a task that took them 7 days, utilizing what she described as the "best in class" tools available. "From a food safety perspective," she emphasized, "if there is a recall, those 7 days are significant." After the block chain technology was piloted, she reported, the mango package test was repeated. This time, utilizing the block chain technology, it took the team only 2.2 seconds to identify a farm in Mexico as the origin of the mangoes. The lesson, Denniston said, is not that block chain technology is "the answer," because in fact, questions remain about its scale and application, and work is still under way with suppliers on determining how to utilize the technology. Rather, she asserted, the lesson is the importance of considering ways to innovate with respect to collecting this kind of information.

Engage the People Who Are Impacted by the Issues

Denniston observed that although the fourth lesson—engage the people who are impacted by the issues—seems self-explanatory, it had been the subject of little discussion at this workshop. In fact, she included it as a lesson learned not because Walmart does this particularly well, but because the company has noticed its lack. As an example, she pointed out that the major tools Walmart uses in its efforts to combat deforestation include market signals and government responses; however, a community that may not have an economically viable alternative and that is trying to survive and feed its families does not care about market signals or government regulations. "If we don't get to know what assets that community has as an alternative," she stressed, "we won't be successful."

Economics Help Drive Innovation

According to Denniston, one way to articulate the fifth lesson—that economics help drive innovation—is that if there is a strong enough business case for an idea, people will figure out how to implement it. As an example, Walmart set a goal of sending zero food waste to landfills, but had no idea how to accomplish this. However, Denniston reported, food waste is expensive, so determining how to eliminate it became an economic imperative. Over the past couple of years, she noted, the company has been testing ways to reduce food waste from strawberries. Through a series of iterative experiments, it has successfully removed about a day and a half from the supply chain, extended the freshness life of the product by 2 to 3 days, and increased by 70 percent the amount of strawberries out on the floor in stores rather than sitting in warehouses. Denniston added that Walmart also invests heavily in food recovery, and in 2017 donated about 750 million pounds of food to people in need.

Consumer Engagement Helps Drive Demand

In describing the sixth lesson learned—that consumer engagement helps drive demand—Denniston observed that it is difficult to create consumer demand. It is not something a retailer can decide to do, she pointed out, but it is something a retailer can signal. So, for example, when Walmart made its healthier food commitments in 2011, it not only reformulated products by reducing sugar and sodium and removing trans fats altogether, but also introduced an icon to help consumers with decision making. Specifically, Denniston recounted, the company introduced a "best if used by" date to help consumers avoid confusion regarding expiration dates that do not specify "sell by" or "use by." She explained that the new icon is now on 92 percent of Walmart's private-label brands in the United States. According to Denniston, this one small change has eliminated an estimated 660 million pounds of food waste, and she described this kind of tool as one with a great deal of promise. In her opinion, it is critically important that greater consideration be given to how to shift some of the signaling and deliver sustainability guidance in a more tailored, systematic way.

Questions to Consider

Denniston concluded by offering three questions to consider. First, what really needs to happen? What does a sustainable food system look like? Second, why isn't it happening? How can the people who are actually making sustainable food choices every day be engaged? What are the frictions? What are the barriers? Lastly, she asked, "What would have to be different tomorrow for us to get that system that we are looking for?" How can people be provided the tools and guidance needed to shift behavior?

DISCUSSION

Following Denniston's presentation, she, Blackstone, Heller, and Mitloehner participated in an open discussion with the audience, summarized here.

Environmental Impact of Transportation: Nutrient-Dense Versus Energy-Dense Food Supply Chains

Imagine a city of 20 million people, each of whom is eating a diet of 2,000 calories, Drewnowski proposed. Further suppose that the average energy density of their diets, filled with broccoli, leafy greens, baby carrots, and other vegetables, is one-half calorie per gram. That, Drewnowski said, amounts to about 80,000 to 100,000 tons of food moving through the city streets every day to be delivered to people, depending on how much is lost to waste. But if that same population were to switch to a diet filled with processed foods or ultra-processed foods, such as chocolate and potato chips, with an average energy density of 5 calories per gram, only about 8,000 tons of food would be moving through the city streets every day. As a result, transportation costs would be cut by one-tenth. Plus, Drewnowski added, energy-dense foods are cheaper. He asked what these observations mean in terms of how a shift toward a less energy-dense diet would play out economically in the long term. "My fear," he said, "is that for big cities, many of them poor, there are going to be incredible economic pressures to eat energy-dense diets which are cheap but nutrient poor."

Blackstone replied by reiterating that focusing overly on food miles is unwarranted, as the associated environmental impact does not compare with the impacts of production. That said, she added, there are differences in transportation efficiency, noting that the difference in transportation impact between a fruit and vegetable supply chain and a processed food supply chain depends on how the foods are transported. If the same fruits and vegetables are being air-freighted, she pointed out, their transportation will have a much larger environmental impact—by an order of magnitude—than if they are being transported by trucks. Alternatively, if they are being transported on fully loaded trucks, the difference is not as dramatic as an order of magnitude.

Comparing Greenhouse Gas Emissions: By Calories or Weight?

"We don't carry food," Drewnowski observed. "We eat it." Moreover, while there are no requirements for any particular weight of food to be consumed daily, there are requirements for calories (approximately 2,000) and nutrients. He asked, then, why GHG emissions are measured per kilogram of food (as Heller had done during his presentation) when examining diet and suggested that calories are a more appropriate metric.

Heller explained that he and his colleagues used GHG per kilogram because the intake data they had were by weight. He considered the metric merely an avenue for linking GHG emissions and intake and agreed that it is not the best metric for comparing different foods. But in his opinion, neither is caloric content. Using calories as a metric, he argued, leads to such situations as lettuce having a greater GHG emissions impact than pork. "And that's fairly illogical as well," he asserted.

Blackstone agreed with Drewnowski that in the context of a diet pattern, it makes sense to use a calorie comparison. In a healthy diet, she observed, one consumes a much smaller quantity of calories from fruits and vegetables relative to other foods. But like Heller, she disagreed with Drewnowski about the use of calories at the level of individual foods. "It skews," she argued.

Consequences of China's One-Child Versus Two-Child Policies

When asked by an audience member about the environmental impact of China's two-child policy compared with its one-child policy, Mitloehner replied that the lifting of the one-child policy in China will not make a great difference because the vast majority of families will continue to have only one child—the expense of raising a larger family is too great. He believes that, more than the number of children per family, increasing life expectancy is what is driving the population structure of China. He pointed out that the average Chinese individual lives much longer today than was the case 20 to 30 years ago, which cumulatively has had a large effect on the country's total population density.

Environmental Impact of Different Breeds of Livestock

When asked by Regina Tan, USDA, whether different livestock breeds—for example, Jersey versus Holstein cows—have different environmental impacts and whether there has been any international effort to share breeding stock, Mitloehner replied that in general, yes, there are significant differences among breeds. For example, a smaller-framed Jersey is more efficient at producing milk relative to a larger-framed Holstein. He agreed about the need to trade livestock internationally to improve breeds, but cautioned that breeds also need to be adapted to local conditions.

Improving the Infrastructure of Veterinary Medicine

Tan also asked whether there have been international efforts to improve the infrastructure of veterinary medicine. Mitloehner replied that the veterinary infrastructure is largely underdeveloped in much of the developing world, where livestock are often infested with parasites that consume the nutrients intended for them. This is a "grave concern," he said, because the animals are often not vaccinated or otherwise treated appropriately. He pointed out that this leads to enormous production losses, which in turn drive environmental impact. In his opinion, the question is, "Are we ready for a new green revolution?"

Disclosing Conflicts of Interest

Lurie proposed that a standard policy of the Food Forum be for all speakers to disclose their conflicts of interest, and that this policy be implemented immediately. Noting that on this panel, Denniston and Heller had been quite clear about their conflicts of interest, he asked Mitloehner and Blackstone whether they had any conflicts they would like to disclose.

Mitloehner disclosed that about 98 percent of his funding comes from public sources, including EPA and the California Air Resources Board, and that the remaining 2 percent comes from companies that fund technology research on the mitigation of emissions. As an example of the latter, he mentioned pharmaceutical companies at the forefront of developing technologies that help reduce environmental footprints (e.g., feed additives that reduce GHG emissions). Blackstone disclosed that her funding comes entirely from her academic institution and an environmental leadership foundation.

Are Dietary Shifts Enough to Move the Needle on Climate Change?

Jackie Schulz, Kraft Heinz, Glenview, Illinois, informed the audience that she had recently attended the Institute of Food Technologists' (IFT's) annual meeting, where she saw Dennis Dimick's presentation "Eyes on Earth." In line with that presentation, she commented on the urgency of the climate change crisis. She asked the panel to reflect on whether dietary shifts, which obviously have potential benefits, are enough to move the needle on climate change as quickly as is needed, and whether reductions in fossil fuel use and food waste would have a greater impact more quickly.

Mitloehner replied that in his opinion, dietary changes will occur, but they will occur slowly. Moreover, he suggested, many parts of the world will see shifts toward, not away from, a more animal-based diet. Re-educating those masses of people will take a long time, he argued, "time that we don't have." He clarified that he did not mean to imply that this re-education should not happen, but that a direct, major change in carbon emissions is needed. He reiterated that the vast majority of carbon emissions is driven by fossil fuel use. "That is undisputed internationally, I believe," he said. The biggest players, he pointed out, are countries such as China and India that currently are mounting a large drive to electrify their vehicle fleets. According to Mitloehner, "that will have a profound impact." In the United States, he added, "what we drive" and "how we heat or cool our houses" also has a profound impact. He was adamant that food choices not be compared with fossil fuel choices. "There is no comparison between these two," he stressed, "particularly in a country like this one."

The Environmental Impact of Beef Consumption: Conflicting Perspectives

Regarding the production efficiency of dietary shifts, an audience member observed that on the first day of the workshop (summarized in Chapters 2 through 4), many speakers had expressed "a beef with beef," that is, the view that beef is a big problem with respect to GHG emissions and land use. Today, in contrast, Mitloehner had remarked that beef accounts for only 4 percent of U.S. GHG emissions and implied that beef consumption in the United States is not a concern. According to this audience member, the reason estimates of U.S. GHG emissions from beef are so low is that use of pasture land use is assumed to be free from a GHG perspective. In addition, she asserted that it is important to view the environmental impact of beef consumption from a system point of view: that 3 billion people are going to enter the global middle class and that dairy and beef consumption are going to increase by 70 to 80 percent. Because all pasture lands worldwide are being used currently but many are not being used productively, she agreed with Mitloehner that investing in livestock productivity is essential. But even with that investment and even if livestock productivity worldwide were raised to U.S. levels, she stressed, it still would not be possible to meet the expected 70 to 80 percent increase in demand for beef. That growing demand, she pointed out, will continue to drive deforestation. Thus, she concluded, "it is really important in high beef consumption countries, like the U.S., the UK, and others, that we have reductions in order to allow others to eat beef as they enter the global middle class."

Mitloehner clarified that the 4 percent figure for the United States was for all livestock, not just beef, and that it referred only to direct emissions. Still, he acknowledged, beef alone is no doubt an important driver of GHG emissions. He also agreed that the increased demand for beef will be significant globally. In his opinion, however, one of the most salient aspects of the carbon footprint of beef globally is the extreme inefficiency of beef production in much of the developing world. He explained that while a beef steer in the United States is "finished" at 14 months of age, that animal peer in Africa may live 10, 15, or 20 years before being harvested. For Mitloehner, addressing these inefficiencies is important to reduce the global carbon footprint of livestock.

Elaborating on the equity perspective, Blackstone remarked that, even if GHG emissions due to livestock in the United States are only 5.5 percent of total U.S. GHG emissions, they are in fact massive and probably greater than those in many other countries. In addition, she argued, because the United States has been emitting such large amounts of GHGs for so long, the nation has an ethical obligation to reduce its emissions regardless of breakdown by sector.

Given the urgency of the climate change crisis, Heller opined that no single sector is going to solve the problem. Rather, he argued, efforts are needed on all fronts.

Consumption-Based Greenhouse Gas Emissions

Springmann commented on the push internationally to examine GHG emissions from a consumption-based perspective. He mentioned as an example work being done by the Center for International Climate Research (CICERO) in Norway (Barrett et al., 2013). Mitloehner added that, while many researchers do look at consumption-based emissions as an academic exercise, the GHG emission inventories of EPA are prepared using a production-based approach.

Promoting Local and Regional Food Systems to Consumers: Any Federal Policies?

Rebecca Boehm, University of Connecticut, pointed to the recent farm bill negotiations, in which programs that supported local food systems, such as the Food Insecurity Nutrition Incentive Grant program, received more funding and garnered bipartisan support. She wondered whether there were any federal policies in place to promote local and regional food systems to consumers in an effort to drive demand for such systems, such as through the DGA.

Blackstone commented that, while redemption of Supplemental Nutrition Assistance Program (SNAP) vouchers at farmers' markets has been increasing over time because of the portals provided where people can use their electronic benefits transfer (EBT) cards, the company that handles all of these EBT transfers is ceasing operations. She cautioned that many farmers' markets will then be unable to process SNAP vouchers, and stressed the importance of finding some way to continue support for a highly successful program that provides access to healthy foods in low-income communities.

6

Concluding Discussion

In the concluding session of the workshop, moderated by Erik Olson, Natural Resources Defense Council, Washington, DC, five previous speakers or moderators participated in a panel discussion: Adam Drewnowski, Jessica Fanzo, Diego Rose, Marco Springmann, and David Tilman. The session opened with Olson asking the panelists to reflect on the workshop and share their takeaways. He then described a hypothetical future scenario involving a meeting in the White House and asked each panelist to imagine him- or herself as the Czar of Sustainable Foods. He asked the panelists what they would say to each of the other people present at the meeting (the President, Bill Gates, and the chief executive officer [CEO] of Walmart). The session ended with an open discussion with the audience. This chapter summarizes the information and opinions that emerged during this session.

OVERALL IMPRESSIONS AND TAKEAWAYS

The Overwhelming Nature of the Data, the Complexity of the Science, But Promising Steps Forward

Fanzo commented on the rich conversations that had taken place over the course of the workshop and the many different perspectives from science and the private sector they reflected. She noted, however, a gap in representation from government and policy makers and the need for more voices from the social sciences. She also found the data to be a bit overwhelming, while acknowledging that this is an inevitable result of the complexity of working in such a multidisciplinary space. Reflecting on the controversy surrounding the Food and Agriculture Organization (FAO) report *Livestock's Long Shadow: Environmental Issues and Options* (FAO, 2006), she described how someone without expertise in a particular area can "go down a rabbit hole" and believe that the content of whatever he or she is reading is robust, whether it is or not. Given the difficulty that even she has in interpreting climate data, she imagined that it must be extremely difficult for consumers, producers, and policy makers to "weed through" and make sense of the science. She observed further that some people believe what is in the FAO (2006) report, while others are very critical, depending on their perspectives, incentives, and funding. Context always matters, she stressed.

At the same time, given the many minds being brought together to address sustainability, Fanzo expressed hope. Using the United Nations (UN) Sustainable Development Goals (SDGs) as a framework and having conversations such as those at this workshop is, she argued, "a promising step compared to where we were 5, 10 years ago."

Equity, Trade-Offs, and Unanswered Questions

Tilman identified the issue of equity as a recurring theme over the course of the workshop. In his opinion, the world will be stable in the long term only if greater equity exists among individuals both within and across societies. He observed that the poorest countries are now among those with the highest economic growth rates; thus, 50 to 100 years from now, there will be much greater economic equity among countries. But there will be a cost to that equity, he asserted, because of the greater per capita environmental impacts that richer individuals tend to create. Diet has major implications for human health, he added, but asked what the environmental impacts will be of people worldwide living longer, healthier lives, with lower morbidity and mortality rates.

Tilman also was bothered by some of the comments about relative greenhouse gas (GHG) emissions among nations. For him, the question is, "What do we on average, as a citizen of Earth, have the right to do if we are going to have a world that is really equitable and sustainable in the long term?"

While Tilman acknowledged not having answers to these questions, he believes much of the change needed is behavioral. For him, the most difficult question is how to come to grips with the various costs and benefits of how people live and how they agree as individuals, as nations, and globally about choices around foods, energy, land, water quality, and other issues related to sustainable diets. He expressed his hope that there is still time for rational thought and change. "It's not a freight train about to hit a wall," he acknowledged. Nonetheless, he argued, sustainable life on Earth not just 10 years from now, but 1,000 and 10,000 years from now, will require a multidisciplinary, multicultural approach that recognizes global interdependence.

Shifting Toward More Plant-Based Eating

Springmann agreed with Fanzo's and Tilman's remarks about the need for multiple perspectives. However, he did not find the data overwhelming or the questions unanswerable. For him, looking at different perspectives actually helps reduce confusion and clarify direction. He explained that the basic factor underlying the differential environmental footprints of animal- and plant-based foods is the feed conversion ratio; that is, it always takes more feed to feed animals than if humans were to eat the feed themselves. He remarked on the extensive discussion during the workshop, particularly in the last session (summarized in Chapter 5), on GHG emissions associated with different diets. But he stressed that it is also clear that if people in high meat-consuming countries were to eat less meat, especially less red and processed meat, large health benefits would result, citing as an example that there is a possible mechanistic explanation for an association between red meat, for example, and colorectal cancer. Thus, he summarized, there are benefits in both dimensions—environmental and human health. He added that plant-based foods in general are known to be cheaper—perhaps not in supermarkets such as Whole Foods where plant-based foods are marketed to a specific demographic, but generally from a production perspective. The challenge, he asserted, is how to structure the food system to make those foods available. Overall, he argued, a dietary change toward a more sustainable diet probably means a shift toward a more plant-based diet.

Springmann clarified that this observation does not necessarily mean that everyone needs to become vegan; rather, it means a shift toward plant-based eating. The challenge, he suggested, is how. He referred to Ranganathan's presentation (summarized in Chapter 4) on lessons learned from private-sector marketing on how to shift behavior. He speculated that it is probably unrealistic to expect people to eliminate meat from their diets entirely, but it is more likely that some people would eat vegan for a certain amount of time each week. He encouraged the retail sector to provide plant-based products so that people would have that choice, stating that if people ate red or processed meat only once per week, for example, the world would probably be much more sustainable.

The Complexity of Sustainable Food Systems, the Challenge of Obtaining Good-Quality Data, and the Issue of Health Equity

The first takeaway for Drewnowksi was that sustainable food systems are complicated, multisectoral, and transdisciplinary and that achieving sustainability will require the involvement of a range of expertise, from social science to epidemiology to the food industry. For him, it is helpful to revisit the FAO definition of a sustainable diet and its four domains: (1) health and nutrition, (2) economics, (3) society, and (4) the environment. Thus, he stressed, the environment is only one of several domains of a sustainable diet, and he urged greater consideration of the broader picture and other parts of that picture, from affordability to labor issues to health equity. In his opinion, focusing only on the environment can be misleading, especially since the environmental context is so different from one country or geography to another—even within the United States. Globally, he pointed out, there are differences not only in context, but also in the quality of environmental data.

Indeed, the need for good-quality data was a second take-home message for Drewnowski. Referring to Afshin's presentation on the health metric, consumption, and other data that the Global Burden of Disease (GBD) project is combining, coding, and converting into models (see Chapter 3), he commented on the complexity of understanding even where dietary data are and sustainable diets based on those data can be modeled. In Drewnowski's opinion, while GBD has been extremely expensive, it is "money well spent," given that it has created the best picture available of the global burden of disease.

A third takeaway for Drewnowski was the issue of health equity. There is no standard diet, he asserted; rather, different people consume different diets with different costs. He mentioned again that in Seattle, he has observed differences in obesity rates on the order of 600 percent based simply on where people live—a socioeconomic difference that dwarfs any kind of difference by race, ethnicity, age, sex, or any other factor. He encouraged workshop participants to keep in mind the issue of diet disparity and health equity.

Providing Sustainable Diet Guidance, Understanding What Drives Individual Behavior, and Communicating Among Disciplines

Rose drew a parallel between the workshop discussion on sustainable diets and the dietary guidance process in the United States. He explained that in the late 1970s, before the first *Dietary Guidelines for Americans* (DGA) was issued in 1980, the U.S. Senate issued a set of dietary guidelines called *The Dietary Goals for the United States*. That senators were promulgating guidelines prompted the nutrition community, as well as the legislative community, to call for the involvement of professionals. In Rose's opinion, one of the wise decisions made when the first DGA was issued was to revisit the guidelines every 5 years. Thus, he observed, experts can communicate to the public what is understood based on the best available science, knowing there will be an opportunity in another 5 years to revise their recommendations. "I think we are sort of at that point here with sustainable diets," he suggested. Much is known and can be communicated to the public and policy makers now, and this information can be revisited in 4 to 5 years to see whether any changes should be made to the advice offered.

Another takeaway for Rose was the importance of modeling at the individual level, given that it is individuals who make decisions about what to eat (as described in Heller's presentation, summarized in Chapter 5, on their joint work in linking environmental impacts to National Health and Nutrition Examination Survey [NHANES] dietary data). "That is where the change happens," Rose asserted. If the goal is to move people toward less waste and a more plant-based diet, he elaborated, it is important to know what motivates individuals. Thus, he called for a greater focus on drivers of individual-level change, noting that Ranganathan had described some of these drivers in her presentation (summarized in Chapter 4). He added that, although there had been little discussion about social media at the workshop, they are known to be a powerful driver of behavioral change and are used a great deal in marketing. "I think we need to tap more into that," he said. Thus, he echoed calls to expand expertise at the next workshop on sustainable diets to include more social scientists, including sociologists, anthropologists, and economists, as well as marketing experts. Because policies and the food environment are also important drivers of change, he argued further for political scientists and politicians to be present in future discussions to enable a better understanding of how politicians perceive the world and what political drivers can create the will to make the necessary changes.

Finally, Rose stressed that having all of these different people in the room will require getting better at interdisciplinary communication. He mentioned that in his own work, Heller is an example of someone from another discipline with whom he has resolved language issues, differences in publication style, differences in how data are handled, and other challenges, and he suspects that anyone working as part of an interdisciplinary team has had a similar experience. "I think it is a challenge that we need to keep pursuing," he said, "because that is how we are really going to get to a better conclusion."

A HYPOTHETICAL SCENARIO: WHAT WOULD YOU SAY?

Olson asked the panelists to imagine a hypothetical future scenario in which a new President has just been inaugurated, and "you," the panelist, have been invited to the White House as the Czar of Sustainable Foods to meet with three people: (1) the President, who wants to hear what you, the new Czar of Sustainable Foods, have to say; (2) Bill Gates, who is going to give money to nongovernmental organizations (NGOs) to do whatever he wants them to do; and (3) the CEO of Walmart. You are each allowed two sentences, he instructed the panelists, to tell each of these three people the number one thing they should do.

Drewnowski began. He offered that he would say to the President that the major problems with diet quality are related to income and socioeconomic status and that the "first order of the day" is redistribution of income. To Bill Gates, he would call for accountability. He would tell Gates that it is time to step away from foundations that are not accountable to anyone and to restore functions formerly served by FAO, the World Health Organization (WHO), and government institutions. To the CEO of Walmart, he quipped, "I would say, 'What are you doing about Amazon?'"

For Springmann, the number one thing he would ask of the President would be to eliminate what he characterized as the "crazy" dairy recommendations in the DGA. He referred to results from Heller's research showing the role of dairy in nonsustainable diets (see Figure 5-4 in Chapter 5). He would also ask the President to revise the U.S. calcium recommendations, as they underpin the dairy recommendations. As for Gates, Springmann agreed with Drewnowski's response. In addition, he would ask Gates to rethink official development aid, for example, and instead of investing in specific food groups, think about how to develop sustainable food systems holistically in developing countries. He would suggest that Gates perhaps engage Walmart's help in cold chain logistics. And he would suggest to the Walmart CEO that the company think more about food groups and their role in sustainable diets.

Tilman would encourage the President to choose a cabinet and cabinet secretaries based on their ability and desire to advance a science-based agenda throughout government. He expressed his view that "with a science-based agenda, we can address many of the problems that this group has been discussing." He would encourage the Walmart CEO to find ways to package and sell foods that reduce waste at the consumer level. In addition, he would request that Walmart use its marketing skills to encourage consumers to purchase more fruits and vegetables. To Gates, he would request money for a Nobel-like prize for developing and popularizing the best tasting, healthiest foods possible. Each year, the winners would be chosen based on an international contest with a highly publicized televised cook-off.

Fanzo would ask the President to commit to the SDGs and to hold the United States accountable for attempting to achieve those goals. She would ask Gates to invest more in nutrition. According to Fanzo, Gates has historically not been convinced of the case for nutrition, particularly undernutrition, and the current portfolio for nutrition of the Bill & Melinda Gates Foundation is very small compared with health or even agriculture development. "I would present the case to him that diets are incredibly important," she said. Acknowledging the impossibility of such a request, she would say to the Walmart CEO, "Stop selling junk food." She would suggest that Walmart be the first retailer not to have any junk food in its stores. "Wouldn't that be amazing?" she asked.

To the President, Rose would argue the importance of sustainable diets, particularly with respect to climate change, and he would point out the many tools in the President's administration available for addressing this issue (e.g., guidelines, food labeling, taxes). Like Fanzo, he would encourage Gates to increase the foundation's nutrition portfolio. Also like Fanzo, he would urge the Walmart CEO to reduce the sale of junk food. In addition, he would urge Walmart to reduce food waste and, more generally, commit to sustainable foods.

QUESTIONS FROM THE AUDIENCE

Different Approaches to Analyzing and Interpreting Data on Sustainable Diets

Tahiri agreed with Fanzo's remarks about the overwhelming nature of data on sustainable diets. For her, it is as though everyone is climbing the same mountain, but from different angles. She finds this to be especially true with respect to modeling the population effects of changes in meat consumption. She asked whether it is possible to consolidate all the different datasets that had been examined over the course of the workshop.

Springmann countered that the different perspectives and multiple data sources discussed throughout the workshop are not to be discouraged. He described the data as "imperfect descriptions of reality." So in his opinion, the more sources there are, the better—one can then ask the same question of the different sources to see if they agree.

Rose added that in a way, a convergence has already taken place. He mentioned results from the models Springmann had described (summarized in Chapter 4) converging with results from the individual-level study described by Heller (summarized in Chapter 5). "Basically we are seeing some of the same patterns," Rose said, including that food waste and beef and dairy are driving many of the environmental impacts of the food system.

The Four Dimensions of Sustainable Diets

Tahiri expressed concern that the focus on the environmental dimension of sustainable diets and the failure to consider the other three components (health and nutrition, economics, and society) is worse than misleading, as Drewnowski had observed. In her opinion, if health, affordability, and accessibility are not taken into account, it will be impossible to convince consumers and others who need to be convinced to do what is necessary to advance sustainable diets. She observed that there had been little discussion during the workshop about how to be an ambassador for all four components of sustainability, not just the environmental component.

Drewnowski referred to Tilman's idea of a "great cook-off" to find a food that is nutrient-rich and also affordable, appealing, and planet-friendly. "What is that food?" he asked. He agreed that affordability in particular is of utmost concern, as it "goes to the heart of health equity."

Related to these other dimensions of sustainability, an audience member suggested that perhaps another workshop should be planned to focus on the economic impacts of the dietary transitions that had been discussed at this workshop. She expressed particular interest in the impacts on farmers' incomes in developing countries, but also in developed countries, given that 28 percent of the global workforce is in this sector. If farmers do not earn a decent living, she argued, they will be unable to invest in the productivity increases needed to reduce the environmental impact of agriculture.

Fanzo agreed that this would be a great workshop idea, calling attention to a recent *Lancet* series on the economics of noncommunicable diseases. "I think we need the same thing," Fanzo said, but on the economics of nutrition outcomes.

Breaking Down Silos and Thinking More Holistically

Kate Houston of Cargill, Inc., suggested that part of the challenge to addressing all four components of sustainable diets is that everyone acknowledges the components' equal importance, yet, she said, "we get so siloed in our work." She added that this is the case even in companies, where experts are working to solve different elements of a broader challenge. She asked the panelists for suggestions on how to break these silos down and encourage different parts of the academic community and the private sector to think more holistically about the issues and solutions.

Tilman responded that, based on his experience, the only way to get people with different backgrounds to collaborate is to gather them in the same place. Architecture or geography, he said, "ends up being intellectual destiny." He described how at his university, he had a math professor across the hall from him, an economist down the hall, and a historian neighbor as well. He encouraged finding such opportunities to enable regular interaction. He added that in many disciplines, working groups are formed when some sort of formal funding mechanism brings people together four or five times per year. A similar working group encompassing the diversity represented at this workshop could make great progress, he asserted. He cautioned, however, that the first few meetings would be dedicated to simply finding out how to communicate effectively.

Building on Tilman's response, Fanzo observed that there are many ways to think about "place." She suggested that the global framework of the SDGs is another type of place, one where the world has been meeting and where a universal framework of action around sustainable development for the next 15 years has been constructed. She stressed not only that the development of the SDGs brought every country to the table, but also that the agreement reached was more collective than was the case for the Millennium Development Goals, with donors really rallying behind the SDGs. Now, she noted, countries are making their own SDG plans, but with different priorities. For example, Nepal, being a land-locked country, is not focusing as intensely on the SDG related to life under water. Countries also are basing their priorities on what they can feasibly do within the next 10 years. According to Fanzo, however, almost every country has prioritized SDG 2: end hunger, achieve food security and improved nutrition, and promote sustainable agriculture.

Drewnowski suggested yet another strategy for breaking down silos, one that operates at what he described as a micro level. He reported that the University of Washington recently approved an undergraduate major in food systems, to be administered by the School of Public Health in collaboration with the School of Business, the School of Law, the College of Engineering, the College of the Environment, and the College of Built Environments. The new major is serving as a mechanism for bringing people from different disciplines and sectors together, in some cases for the first time, all working toward population health. Drewnowski is hoping that the faculty from these different schools and colleges will come together initially to talk about the undergraduate curriculum, but eventually will discuss research and joint projects and grants.

Rose added that beyond finding ways to work together either in a place or on a specific project, as Fanzo and Tilman had discussed, or ways to study together, as Drewnowski had described, it is also important to convey the need for a certain humility to students—that what they study or what they know is not everything. It is vital, he stressed, for students to understand that there are important issues beyond their disciplinary knowledge and that they need to respect other people's disciplines and talents.

In addition, Rose emphasized the importance of not just working together but also playing together if people are to get along with one another.

As an example, he cited dinners or receptions after workshops such as this, where people have the opportunity to see each other as people, not just professionals. Doing so, he argued, makes it easier to overcome the hurdles that exist in the face of disagreement, misunderstanding, or differing objectives.

Springmann echoed Rose's call for play and added that tolerance is also important. He encouraged talking to one other, asking questions about what drives people in other disciplines or sectors, and being tolerant of different views.

References

Aleksandrowicz, L., R. Green, E. J. Joy, P. Smith, and A. Haines. 2016. The impacts of dietary change on greenhouse gas emissions, land use, water use, and health: A systematic review. *PLoS ONE* 11(11):e0165797.

Alexandratos, N., and J. Bruinsma. 2012. *World agriculture towards 2030/2050. The 2012 revision*. ESA working paper no. 12-03. Rome, Italy: FAO.

Bacon, L., and D. Krpan. 2018. (Not) eating for the environment: The impact of restaurant menu design on vegetarian food choice. *Appetite* 125:190–200. doi: 10.1016/j.appet.2018.02.006.

Bajželj, B., K. S. Richards, J. M. Allwood, P. Smith, J. S. Dennis, E. Curmi, and C. A. Gilligan. 2014. Importance of food-demand management for climate mitigation. *Nature Climate Change* 4:924–929.

Barrett, J., P. Glen, T. Wiedmann, K. Scott, M. Lenzen, K. Roelich, and C. Le Quéré. 2013. Consumption-based GHG emission accounting: A U.K. case study. *Climate Policy* 13(4):451–470.

Beauman, C., G. Cannon, I. Elmadfa, P. Glasauer, I. Hoffmann, M. Keller, M. Krawinkel, T. Lang, C. Leitzmann, B. Lotsch, and B. Margetts. 2005. The Giessen Declaration. *Public Health Nutrition* 8(6A):783–786.

Bennetzen, E. H., P. Smith, and J. R. Porter. 2016. Decoupling of greenhouse gas emissions from global agricultural production: 1970–2050. *Global Change Biology* 22(2):763–781.

Bhutta, Z. A., T. Ahmed, R. E. Black, S. Cousens, K. Dewey, E. Giugliani, B. A. Haider, B. Kirkwood, S. S. Morris, H. P. Sachdev, and M. Shekar. 2008. What works? Interventions for maternal and child undernutrition and survival. *The Lancet* 371(9610):417–440.

Bhutta, Z. A., J. K. Das, J. Rizvi, M. F. Gaffey, N. Walker, S. Horton, P. Webb, A. Lartey, and R. E. Black. 2013. Evidence-based interventions for improvement of maternal and child nutrition: What can be done and at what cost? *Lancet: Nutrition Interventions Review Group and the Maternal and Child Nutrition Study Group* 382(98930):452–477.

Blackstone, N. T. 2018. *Local and regional food systems in sustainable diets*. Presentation, National Academies Workshop, Washington, DC, August 1. http://www.nationalacademies.org/hmd/~/media/Files/Activity%20Files/Nutrition/FoodForum/August%202018/14%20BlackstoneFood%20Forum20180802.pdf (accessed January 21, 2019).

Blackstone, N. T., N. H. El-Abbadi, M. S. McCabe, T. S. Griffin, and M. E. Nelson. 2018. Linking sustainability to the healthy eating patterns of the *Dietary Guidelines for Americans*: A modeling study. *Lancet Planet Health* 2(8):e344–e352.

Boehm, R., P. E. Wilde, M. Ver Ploeg, C. Costello, and S. B. Cash. 2018. A comprehensive life cycle assessment of greenhouse gas emissions from U.S. household food choice. *Food Policy* 79:67–76. doi: 10.1016/j.foodpol.2018.05.004.

Bray, G. A., and B. M. Popkin. 1998. Dietary fat does affect obesity! *American Journal of Clinical Nutrition* 68(6):1157–1173.

Bray, G. A., S. J. Nielsen, and B. M. Popkin. 2004. Consumption of high-fructose corn syrup in beverages may play a role in the epidemic of obesity. *American Journal of Clinical Nutrition* 79(4):537–543.

Bruinsma, J. 2009. The resource outlook to 2050: By how much do land, water and crop yields need to increase by 2050? Conference paper in *How to Feed the World in 2050. Proceedings of a Technical Meeting of Experts*, Rome, Italy, June 24–26, 2009. Rome, Italy: FAO. http://www.fao.org/docrep/012/ak542e/ak542e00.htm (accessed September 25, 2018).

Bryngelsson, D., S. Wirsenius, F. Hedenus, and U. Sonesson. 2016. How can the EU climate targets be met? A combined analysis of technological and demand-side changes in food and agriculture. *Food Policy* 56:152–164. doi: 10.1016/j.foodpol.2015.12.012.

CDFA (California Department of Food and Agriculture). 2018. *California agricultural statistics review, 2016–2017*. https://www.cdfa.ca.gov/Statistics/PDFs/2016-17AgReport.pdf (accessed December 11, 2018).

CFR (Council on Foreign Relations). 2013. *Food price volatility and insecurity*. https://www.cfr.org/backgrounder/food-price-volatility-and-insecurity (accessed December 6, 2018).

Clancy, K., and K. Ruhf. 2010. Is local enough? Some arguments for regional food systems. *Choices* 25(1). http://www.choicesmagazine.org/magazine/article.php?article=114 (accessed September 29, 2018).

Clark, M. A. 2018. *How diets affect human health and environmental sustainability*. Ph.D. dissertation, University of Minnesota. https://conservancy.umn.edu/bitstream/handle/11299/199093/Clark_umn_0130E_19120.pdf?sequence=1&isAllowed=y (accessed December 10, 2018).

CNBC. 2017. *Home food delivery is surging thanks to ease of online ordering, new study shows*. https://www.cnbc.com/2017/07/12/home-food-delivery-is-surging-thanks-to-ease-of-online-ordering-new-study-shows.html (accessed December 6, 2018).

Colasanti, K., J. Hardy, J. Farbman, R. Pirog, J. Fisk, and M. Hamm. 2018. *Findings of the 2017 National Food Hub Survey*. East Lansing, MI: Michigan State University Center for Regional Food Systems & The Wallace Center at Winrock International. http://www.canr.msu.edu/resources/2017-food-hub-survey (accessed September 29, 2018).

Crino, M., G. Sacks, S. Vandevijvere, B. Swinburn, and B. Neal. 2015. The influence on population weight gain and obesity of the macronutrient composition and energy density of the food supply. *Current Obesity Reports* 4(1):1–10.

Crotty, P. 1993. The value of qualitative research in nutrition. *Annual Review of Health Social Sciences* 3(1):109–118.

Davies, P. 2004. Sociology and policy science: Just in time? *The British Journal of Sociology* 55(3):447–450.

de Castro, J. 2000. *Eating behavior: Lessons from the real world of humans*. New York: Elsevier Science. https://pdfs.semanticscholar.org/99b7/13e482dbdc350c8130127f6d701a02a80659.pdf (accessed January 4, 2019).

de Onis, M., M. Blössner, and E. Borghi. 2010. Global prevalence and trends of overweight and obesity among preschool children. *American Journal of Clinical Nutrition* 92(5):1257–1264.

de Onis, M., M. Blössner, and E. Borghi. 2012. Prevalence and trends of stunting among preschool children, 1990–2020. *Public Health Nutrition* 15(1):142–148.

Development Initiatives. 2017. *Global Nutrition Report 2017: Nourishing the SDGs*. Bristol, UK: Development Initiatives.

Dewey, K. G., and B. S. Vitta. 2013. Strategies for ensuring adequate nutrient intake for infants and young children during the period of complementary feeding. *A&T Technical Brief*, Issue 7. Washington, DC: Alive and Thrive.

Diaz, R. J., and R. Rosenberg. 2008. Spreading dead zones and consequences for marine ecosystems. *Science* 321(5891):926–929.

Downs, S. M., A. Payne, and J. Fanzo. 2017. The development and application of a sustainable diets framework for policy analysis: A case study of Nepal. *Food Policy* 70:40–49. doi: 10.1016/j.foodpol.2017.05.005.

Drewnowski, A. 2017. Uses of nutrient profiling to address public health needs: From regulation to reformulation. *Proceedings of the Nutrition Society* 76(3):220–229.

Drewnowski, A., and V. Fulgoni III. 2008. Nutrient profiling of foods: Creating a nutrient-rich food index. *Nutrition Reviews* 66(1):23–39.

Drewnowski, A., and B. M. Popkin. 2009. The nutrition transition: New trends in the global diet. *Nutrition Reviews* 55(2):31–43.

EIA (U.S. Energy Information Administration). 2012. *Annual energy outlook 2012: With projections to 2035*. Washington, DC: EIA. https://www.eia.gov/outlooks/aeo/pdf/0383(2012).pdf (accessed September 18, 2018).

Elliot, C. 2014. Food as people: Teenagers' perspectives on food personalities and implications for healthy eating. *Social Science & Medicine* 121:85–90. doi: 10.1016/j.socscimed.2014.09.044.

EPA (U.S. Environmental Protection Agency). 2012. *Global anthropogenic non-CO_2 greenhouse gas emissions: 1990–2030*. Washington, DC: Office of Atmospheric Programs, Climate Change Division, EPA. https://www.epa.gov/sites/production/files/2016-05/documents/epa_global_nonco2_projections_dec2012.pdf (accessed September 18, 2018).

EPA. 2017. *U.S. greenhouse gas inventory report: 1990–2014*. https://www.epa.gov/ghgemissions/us-greenhouse-gas-inventory-report-1990-2014 (accessed December 21, 2018).

Fanzo, J., S. Downs, Q. E. Marshall, S. de Pee, and M. W. Bloem. 2017. Value chain focus on food and nutrition security. In *Nutrition and health in a developing world*, 3rd ed., edited by S. de Pee, D. Taren, and M. W. Bloem. New York: Springer International Publishing. Pp. 753–770.

FAO (Food and Agriculture Organization). 2006. *Livestock's long shadow: Environmental issues and options*. Rome, Italy: FAO. http://www.fao.org/docrep/010/a0701e/a0701e.pdf (accessed September 12, 2018).

FAO. 2009. *The state of food and agriculture 2009*. Rome, Italy: FAO. http://www.fao.org/3/a-i0680e.pdf (accessed November 9, 2018).

FAO. 2011. *The state of the world's land and water resources for food and agriculture: Managing systems at risk*. Rome, Italy: FAO. http://www.fao.org/docrep/017/i1688e/i1688e.pdf (accessed September 18, 2018).

FAO. 2012a. *Save food: Global initiative on food loss and waste reduction*. Rome, Italy: FAO. http://www.fao.org/save-food/resources/keyfindings/en (accessed January 4, 2019).

FAO. 2012b. *Sustainable diets and biodiversity: Directions and solutions for policy, research and action*. Proceedings of the International Scientific Symposium, Biodiversity and Sustainable Diets United Against Hunger, November 2010, Rome, Italy. http://www.fao.org/docrep/016/i3004e/i3004e.pdf (accessed September 3, 2018).

FAO. 2013a. *The state of food and agriculture 2013*. Rome, Italy: FAO. http://www.fao.org/docrep/018/i3300e/i3300e.pdf (accessed September 10, 2018).

FAO. 2013b. *Tackling climate change through livestock: A global assessment of emissions and mitigation opportunities*. Rome, Italy: FAO. http://www.fao.org/3/a-i3437e.pdf (accessed September 10, 2018).

FAO. 2014. *Developing sustainable food value chains: Guiding principles*. Rome, Italy: FAO. http://www.fao.org/3/a-i3953e.pdf (accessed September 26, 2018).

FAO. 2016. *Environmental performance of animal feeds supply chains: Guidelines for quantification*. Version 1. Rome, Italy: FAO. http://www.fao.org/3/a-i6433e.pdf (accessed September 13, 2018).

FAO. 2017a. *FAOSTAT database*. Rome, Italy: FAO. http://www.fao.org/faostat/en/#home (accessed September 26, 2018).

FAO. 2017b. *How can value chains be shaped to improve nutrition?* Summary of the online consultation no. 138. Rome, Italy: FAO. http://www.fao.org/3/a-i7605e.pdf (accessed September 26, 2018).

FAO, IFAD (International Fund for Agricultural Development), UNICEF (United Nations Children's Fund), WFP (World Food Programme), and WHO (World Health Organization). 2018. *The state of food security and nutrition in the world, 2018*. http://www.fao.org/3/I9553EN/i9553en.pdf (accessed September 24, 2018).

Fischer, C. G., and T. Garnett. 2016. *Plates, pyramids, planet: Developments in national healthy and sustainable dietary guidelines: A state of play assessment*. Rome, Italy, and Oxford, UK: FAO and Food Climate Research Network. http://www.fao.org/3/a-i5640e.pdf (accessed September 27, 2018).

Foley, J. A., R. Defries, G. P. Asner, C. Barford, G. Bonan, S. R. Carpenter, F. S. Chapin, M. T. Coe, G. C. Daily, H. K. Gibbs, J. H. Helkowski, T. Holloway, E. A. Howard, C. J. Kucharik, C. Monfreda, J. A. Patz, I. C. Prentice, N. Ramankutty, and P. K. Snyder. 2005. Global consequences of land use. *Science* 309(5734):570–574.

Folke, C., S. R. Carpenter, B. Walker, M. Scheffer, T. Chapin, and J. Rockström. 2010. Resilience thinking: Integrating resilience, adaptability and transformability. *Ecology and Society* 15(4):20. http://www.ecologyandsociety.org/vol15/iss4/art20 (accessed December 7, 2018).

Froetschel, M. A., C. L. Ross, R. L. Stewart Jr., M. J. Azain, P. Michot, and R. Rekaya. 2014. Nutritional value of ensiled grocery food waste for cattle. *Journal of Animal Science* 92(11):5124–5133.

Garnett, T. 2014. Three perspectives on sustainable food security: Efficiency, demand restraint, food system transformation. What role for life cycle assessment? *Journal of Cleaner Production* 73(15):10–18.

Gerber, P. J., T. Vellinga, C. Opio, and H. Steinfeld. 2011. Productivity gains and greenhouse gas intensity in dairy systems. *Livestock Science* 139:100–108.

Gill, M., P. Smith, and J. M. Wilkinson. 2010. Mitigating climate change: The role of domestic livestock. *Animal* 4(3):323–333.

GLOPAN (Global Panel on Agriculture and Food Systems for Nutrition). 2016. *Food systems and diets: Facing the challenges of the 21st century*. http://glopan.org/sites/default/files/ForesightReport.pdf (accessed September 18, 2018).

Graziose, M. M., and I. Y. H. Ang. 2018. Factors related to fruit and vegetable consumption at lunch among elementary students: A scoping review. *Preventing Chronic Disease* 15:E55. doi: 10.5888/pcd15.170373.

Gunders, D. 2012. *How America is losing up to 40 percent of its food from farm to fork to landfill* (Issue Paper: 12-06-B). Washington, DC: Natural Resources Defense Council. https://www.nrdc.org/sites/default/files/wasted-food-IP.pdf (accessed January 4, 2019)

Gussow, J. D. 1991. *Chicken Little, tomato sauce, and agriculture: Who will produce tomorrow's food?* New York: Bootstrap Press.

Gustafson, D., A. Gutman, W. Leet, A. Drewnowski, J. Fanzo, and J. Ingram. 2016. Seven food system metrics of sustainable nutrition security. *Sustainability* 8(3):196. doi: 10.3390/su8030196.

Hallström, E., A. Carlsson-Kanyama, and P. Börjesson. 2015. Environmental impact of dietary change: A systematic review. *Journal of Cleaner Production* 91(15):1–11.

Hedenus, F., S. Wirsenius, and D. J. A. Johansson. 2014. The importance of reduced meat and dairy consumption for meeting stringent climate change targets. *Climate Change* 134(1-2):79–91.

Heller, M. C., and G. A. Keoleian. 2014a. Greenhouse gas emission estimates of U.S. dietary choices and food loss. *Journal of Industrial Ecology*. doi: 10.1111/jiec.12174.

Heller, M. C., and G. A. Keoleian. 2014b. *Greenhouse gas emission estimates of the U.S. diet: Aligning nutritional recommendations with environmental concerns*. Proceedings of the 9th International Conference LCA of Food, San Francisco, October 8–10.

Heller, M. C., and G. A. Keoleian. 2015. Greenhouse gas emission estimates of U.S. dietary choices and food loss. *Journal of Industrial Ecology* 19(3):391–401. doi: 10.1111/jiec.12174.

Heller, M. C., A. Willits-Smith, R. Meyer, G. A. Keoleian, and D. Rose. 2018. Greenhouse gas emissions and energy use associated with production of individual self-selected U.S. diets. *Environmental Research Letters* 13(4):044004. https://www.ncbi.nlm.nih.gov/pmc/articles/PMC5964346 (accessed September 12, 2018).

HLPE (High Level Panel of Experts on Food Security and Nutrition). 2017. *Nutrition and food systems: A report by the Committee on World Food Security's High Level Panel of Experts on Food Security and Nutrition*. http://www.fao.org/3/a-i7846e.pdf (accessed September 18, 2018).

Holland, K. 2018. What are the 12 leading causes of death in the United States? *Healthline*, November 1. https://www.healthline.com/health/leading-causes-of-death (accessed December 6, 2018).

Houghton, R. A. 2008. Carbon flux to the atmosphere from land-use changes: 1850–2005. *In TRENDS: A Compendium of Data on Global Change*. http://cdiac.ess-dive.lbl.gov/trends/landuse/houghton/houghton (accessed September 18, 2018).

Houghton, R. A., J. I. House, J. Pongratz, G. R. van der Werf, R. S. DeFries, M. C. Hansen, C. Le Quérre, and N. Ramankutty. 2012. Carbon emissions from land use and land-cover change. *Biogeosciences* 9:5125–5142. doi: 10.5194/bg-9-5125-2012.

IEA (International Energy Agency). 2012. *World Energy Outlook 2012*. https://www.iea.org/publications/freepublications/publication/WEO2012_free.pdf (accessed September 18, 2018).

IFPRI (Veolia Water North America and International Food Policy Research Institute). 2011. *Sustaining growth via water productivity: 2030/2050 scenarios*. Washington, DC, and Chicago, IL: IFPRI. http://growingblue.com/wp-content/uploads/2011/05/IFPRI_VEOLIA_STUDY_2011.pdf (accessed January 21, 2019).

Imamura, F., R. Micha, S. Khatibzadeh, S. Fahimi, P. Shi, J. Powles, D. Mozaffarian, and Global Burden of Diseases Nutrition and Chronic Diseases Expert Group (NutriCoDE). 2015. Dietary quality among men and women in 187 countries in 1990 and 2010: A systematic assessment. *Lancet Global Health* 3(3):e132–e142.

Izumi, B. T., C. L. Eckhardt, J. A. Hallman, K. Herro, and D. A. Barberis. 2015. Harvest for Healthy Kids pilot study: Associations between exposure to a farm-to-preschool intervention and willingness to try and liking of target fruits and vegetables among low-income children in Head Start. *Journal of the Academy of Nutrition and Dietetics* 115(12):2003–2013.

Johnson, R., R. A. Aussenberg, and T. Cowan. 2013. *The role of local food systems in U.S. farm policy*. Report R42155. Washington, DC: U.S. Congressional Research Service.

Johnston, J. L., J. C. Fanzo, and B. Cogill. 2014. Understanding sustainable diets: A descriptive analysis of the determinants and processes that influence diets and their impact on health, food security, and environmental sustainability. *Advances in Nutrition* 5(4):418–429.

Joyce, A., S. Dixon, J. Comfort, and J. Hallett. 2012. Reducing the environmental impact of dietary choice: Perspectives from a behavioural and social change approach. *Journal of Environmental and Public Health* 2012:978672. doi: 10.1155/2012/978672.

Khoury, C. K., A. D. Bjorkman, H. Dempewolf, J. Ramirez-Villegas, L. Guarino, A. Jarvis, L. H. Rieseberg, and P. C. Struik. 2014. Increasing homogeneity in global food supplies and the implications for food security. *Proceedings of the National Academy of Sciences of the United States of America* 111(11):4001–4006.

King, R. P., M. S. Hand, G. DiGiacomo, K. Clancy, M. I. Gómez, S. D. Hardesty, L. Lev, and E. W. McLaughlin. 2010. *Comparing the structure, size, and performance of local and mainstream food supply chains*. ERR-99. Washington, DC: U.S. Department of Agriculture, Economic Research Service.

Le Port, A., T. Bernard, M. Hidrobo, O. Birba, R. Rawat, and M. T. Ruel. 2017. Delivery of iron-fortified yoghurt, through a dairy value chain program, increases hemoglobin concentration among children 24 to 59 months old in Northern Senegal: A cluster-randomized control trial. *PLoS ONE* 12(2):e0172198.

Lea, E., and A. Worsley. 2003. Benefits and barriers to the consumption of a vegetarian diet in Australia. *Public Health Nutrition* 6(5):505–511.

Lindquist, E. J., R. D'Annunzio, A. Gerrand, K. MacDicken, F. Achard, R. Beuchle, A. Brink, H. D. Eva, P. Mayaux, J. San-Miguel-Ayanz, and H.-J. Stibig. 2012. *Global forest land-use change 1990–2005*. FAO forestry paper no. 169. Rome, Italy: FAO and JRC (European Commission Joint Research Centre). http://www.fao.org/docrep/017/i3110e/i3110e.pdf (accessed December 7, 2018).

Low, S. A., A. Adalja, E. Beaulieu, N. Key, S. Martinez, A. Perez, K. Ralston, H. Stewart, S. Suttles, S. Vogel, and B. R. B. Jablonski. 2015. *Trends in U.S. local and regional food systems: A report to Congress*. AP-068. Washington, DC: U.S. Department of Agriculture, Economic Research Service.

Lubungu, M. 2017. Factors affecting the livestock herd size among smallholder households in Zambia. *Tropical Animal Health and Production* 49(8):1607–1612.

Macdiarmid, J. 2013. Is a healthy diet an environmentally sustainable diet? *Proceedings of the National Academy of Sciences of the United States of America* 72(1):13–20.

Macdiarmid, J., J. Kyle, G.W. Horgan, J. Loe, C. Fyfe, A. Johnstone, and G. McNeil. 2012. Sustainable diets for the future: Can we contribute to reducing greenhouse gas emissions by eating a healthy diet? *American Journal of Nutrition* 96(3):632–639.

Macdiarmid, J. I., F. Douglas, and J. Campbell. 2016. Eating like there's no tomorrow: Public awareness of the environmental impact of food and reluctance to eat less meat as part of a sustainable diet. *Appetite* 96:487–493. doi: 10.1016/j.appet.2015.10.011.

Macdiarmid, J. I., H. Clark, S. Whybrow, H. de Ruiter, and G. McNeill. 2018. Assessing national nutrition security: The U.K. reliance on imports to meet population energy and nutrient recommendations. *PLoS ONE* 13(2):e0192649.

Mason, P., and T. Lang. 2017. *Sustainable diets. How ecological nutrition can transform consumption and the food system*. London, UK: Routledge.

Mazur, R., D. Nakimbugwe, M. Ugen, H. K. Musoke, and H. Vasanthakaalam. 2009. Enhancing nutritional value and marketability of beans through research and strengthening key value chain stakeholders in Uganda and Rwanda. In *Dry Grain Pulses Collaborative Research Support Program (CRSP): 2009 technical highlights*. Washington, DC: U.S. Agency for International Development. Pp. 14–23.

Mitloehner, F. 2016. *Livestock's contributions to climate change: Facts and fiction* [White paper]. http://cekern.ucanr.edu/files/256942.pdf (accessed January 4, 2019).

NASEM (National Academies of Sciences, Engineering, and Medicine). 2017. *Redesigning the process for establishing the* Dietary Guidelines for Americans. Washington, DC: The National Academies Press. doi: 10.17226/24883.

Nelson, G., M. Rosegrant, J. Koo, R. Robertson, T. Sulser, T. Zhu, C. Ringler, S. Msangi, A. Palazzo, M. Batka, M. Magalhães, R. Valmonte-Santos, M. Ewing, and D. Lee. 2009. *Climate change: Impact on agriculture and costs of adaptation*. doi: 10.2499/0896295354.

Nelson, M. E., M. W. Hamm, F. B. Hu, S. A. Abrams, and T. S. Griffin. 2016. Alignment of healthy dietary patterns and environmental sustainability: A systematic review. *Advances in Nutrition* 7(6):1005–1025.

Nicholson, C. F., X. He, M. I. Gómez, H. O. Gao, and E. Hill. 2015. Environmental and economic impacts of localizing food systems: The case of dairy supply chains in the Northeastern United States. *Environmental Sciences & Technology* 49(20):12005–12014.

Okin, G. S. 2017. Environmental impacts of food consumption by dogs and cats. *PLoS ONE* 12(8):e0181301. doi: 10.1371/journal.pone.0181301.

Payne, C. L. R., P. Scarborough, and L. Cobiac. 2016. Do low-carbon-emission diets lead to higher nutritional quality and positive health outcomes? A systematic review of the literature. *Public Health Nutrition* 19(14):2654–2661.

Peters, C. J., J. Picardy, J. L. Wilkins, T. S. Griffin, G. W. Fick, and A. F. Darrouzet-Nardi. 2016. Carrying capacity of U.S. agricultural land: Ten diet scenarios. *Elementa: Science of the Anthropocene* 4. doi: 10.12952/journal.elementa.000116.

Pew-MacArthur Results First Initiative. 2014. *Evidence-based policymaking: A guide for effective government*. https://www.pewtrusts.org/-/media/assets/2014/11/evidencebasedpolicymakingaguideforeffectivegovernment.pdf (accessed September 19, 2018).

Popp, A., H. Lotze-Campen, and B. Bodirsky. 2010. Food consumption, diet shifts and associated non-CO_2 greenhouse gases from agricultural production. *Global Environmental Change* 20(3):451–462.

Ramankutty, N., A. T. Evan, C. Monfreda, and J. A. Foley. 2008. Farming the planet: 1. Geographic distribution of global agricultural lands in the year 2000. *Global Biogeochemical Cycles* 22(1). doi: 10.1029/2007GB002952.

Ranganathan, J., D. Vennard, R. Waite, B. Lipinski, T. Searchinger, and GLOBAGRI-WRR Model Authors. 2016. *Shifting diets for a sustainable food future*. Washington, DC: World Resources Institute. https://wriorg.s3.amazonaws.com/s3fs-public/Shifting_Diets_for_a_Sustainable_Food_Future_1.pdf (accessed September 19, 2018).

Rich, N. 2018. Losing earth: The decade we almost stopped climate change. *The New York Times*, August 1. https://www.nytimes.com/interactive/2018/08/01/magazine/climate-change-losing-earth.html (accessed December 7, 2018).

Robinson, S., D. Mason-D'Croz, T. Sulser, S. Islam, R. Robertson, T. Zhu, A. Gueneau, G. Pitois, and M. W. Rosegrant. 2015. *The International Model for Policy Analysis of Agricultural Commodities and Trade (IMPACT): Model description for version 3*. Discussion paper 1483. Washington, DC: International Food Policy Research Institute. doi: 10.2139/ssrn.2741234.

Rose, D., M. C. Heller, and C. A. Roberto. 2018. Position of the society for nutrition education and behavior: The importance of including environmental sustainability in dietary guidance. *Journal of Nutrition Education and Behavior* 118(5):913–919.

Roser, M. 2018. *Future population growth.* https://ourworldindata.org/future-population-growth (accessed December 24, 2018).

Smith, M. R., and S. S. Myers. 2018. Impact of anthropogenic CO_2 emissions on global human nutrition. *Nature Climate Change* 8:834–839. doi: 10.1038/s41558-018-0253-3.

Smith, M. R., R. Micha, C. D. Golden, D. Mozaffarian, and S. S. Myers. 2016. Global Expanded Nutrient Supply (GENuS) model: A new method for estimating the global dietary supply of nutrients. *PLoS ONE* 11(1):e0146976.

Springmann, M., H. C. Godfray, M. Rayner, and P. Scarborough. 2016a. Analysis and valuation of the health and climate change cobenefits of dietary change. *Proceedings of the National Academy of Sciences of the United States of America* 113(15):4146–4151.

Springmann, M., D. Mason-D'Croz, S. Robinson, T. Garnett, H. C. Godfray, D. Gollin, M. Rayner, P. Ballon, and P. Scarborough. 2016b. Global and regional health effects of future food production under climate change: A modelling study. *The Lancet* 387(10031):1937–1946.

Springmann, M., K. Wiebe, D. Mason-D'Croz, T. B. Sulser, M. Rayner, and P. Scarborough. 2018. Health and nutritional aspects of sustainable diet strategies and their association with environmental impacts: A global modelling analysis with country-level detail. *The Lancet* 2(10):e451–e461.

Stein, A. J., and M. Qaim. 2007. The human and economic cost of hidden hunger. *Food and Nutrition Bulletin* 28(2):125–134.

Sutcliffe, S., and J. Court. 2005. *Evidence-based policymaking: What is it? How does it work? What relevance for developing countries?* London, UK: Overseas Development Institute.

Tichenor, N. E., C. J. Peters, G. A. Norris, G. Thoma, and T. S. Griffin. 2017. Life cycle environmental consequences of grass-fed and dairy beef productions in the Northeastern United States. *Journal of Cleaner Production* 142(4):1619–1628.

Tilman, D., and M. Clark. 2014. Global diets link environmental sustainability and human health. *Nature* 515(7528):518–522.

Tilman, D., J. Fargione, B. Wolff, C. D'Antonio, A. Dobson, R. Howarth, D. Schindler, W. H. Schlesinger, D. Simberloff, and D. Swackhamer. 2001. Forecasting agriculturally driven global environmental change. *Science* 292(5515):281–284.

Tilman, D., C. Balzer, J. Hill, and B. L. Befort. 2011. Global food demand and the sustainable intensification of agriculture. *Proceedings of the National Academy of Sciences of the United States of America* 108(50):20260–20264.

Tilman, D., M. Clark, D. R. Williams, K. Kimmel, S. Polasky, and C. Packer. 2017. Future threats to biodiversity and pathways to their prevention. *Nature* 546(7656):73–81.

Tom, M. S., P. S. Fischbeck, and C. T. Hendrickson. 2016. Energy use, blue water footprint, and greenhouse gas emissions for current food consumption patterns and dietary recommendations in the U.S. *Environmental Systems & Decisions* 36(1):92–103.

Turnwald, B. P., D. Z. Boles, and A. J. Crum. 2017. Association between indulgent descriptions and vegetable consumption: Twisted carrots and dynamite beets. *Journal of the American Medical Association Internal Medicine* 177(8):1216–1218.

UC (University of California) Agricultural Issues Center. 2009. *The measure of California agriculture.* http://aic.ucdavis.edu/publications/moca/moca09/moca09_forematter.pdf (accessed December 21, 2018).

UNDESA (United Nations Department of Economic and Social Affairs). 2014. *World urbanization prospects: The 2014 revision, highlights* (ST/ESA/SER.A/352). https://www.compassion.com/multimedia/world-urbanization-prospects.pdf (accessed December 6, 2018).

UNDESA. 2017. *World population prospects: The 2017 revision, key findings and advance tables.* https://esa.un.org/unpd/wpp/publications/files/wpp2017_keyfindings.pdf (accessed September 18, 2018).

USDA (U.S. Department of Agriculture). 2018. *Long-term agricultural projections.* https://www.usda.gov/oce/commodity/projections (accessed December 6, 2018).

Vermeulen, S. J., B. M. Campbell, and J. S. I. Ingram. 2012. Climate change and food systems. *Annual Review of Environment and Resources* 37:195–222. doi: 10.1146/annurev-environ-020411-130608.

Vitousek, P. M., H. A. Mooney, J. Lubchenco, and J. M. Melillo. 1997. Human domination of Earth's ecosystems. *Science* 277(5325):494–499.

Wang, T. 2006. *China—pork powerhouse of the world.* Beijing, China: China Agricultural University, Jinnai Agribusiness Research Center.

Webb, P., and E. Kennedy. 2014. Impacts of agriculture on nutrition: Nature of the evidence and research gaps. *Food and Nutrition Bulletin* 35(1):126–132.

WHO (World Health Organization). 2009. *Global health risks: Mortality and burden of disease attributable to selected major risks.* Geneva, Switzerland: WHO.

WHO and FAO. 1998. *Preparation and use of food-based dietary guidelines.* WHO Technical Report Series. Geneva, Switzerland: WHO.

Wiggins, S., and S. Keats. 2014. *Future diets: Implications for agriculture and food prices.* London, UK: Overseas Development Institute. https://www.odi.org/sites/odi.org.uk/files/odi-assets/publications-opinion-files/8776.pdf (accessed September 19, 2018).

Wilde, P. 2015. Running out of food. *Journal of Health Affairs* 34(11). doi: 10.1377/hlthaff.2015.1130.

Wood, S. A., M. R. Smith, J. Fanzo, R. Remans, and R. S. DeFries. 2018. Trade and the equitability of global food nutrient distribution. *Nature Sustainability* 1:34–37.

World Bank and IHME (Institute for Health Metrics and Evaluation). 2016. *The cost of air pollution.* Washington, DC: World Bank.

WWAP (World Water Assessment Programme). 2012. *Managing water under uncertainty and risk.* United Nations World Water Development Report 4 (Vol. 1). Paris, France: United Nations Educational, Scientific and Cultural Organization. http://www.unesco.org/new/fileadmin/MULTIMEDIA/HQ/SC/pdf/WWDR4%20Volume%201-Managing%20Water%20under%20Uncertainty%20and%20Risk.pdf (accessed December 7, 2018).

Young, E., and L. Quinn. 2002. *Writing effective public policy papers: A guide for policy advisors in Central and Eastern Europe.* Budapest, Hungary: Open Society Institute.

A

Workshop Agenda

SUSTAINABLE DIETS, FOOD, AND NUTRITION: A WORKSHOP

August 1–2, 2018

National Academy of Sciences Building, Lecture Room
2101 Constitution Avenue, NW, Washington, DC

DAY 1, AUGUST 1, 9:00 AM–4:00 PM

9:00 AM	**Welcome and Opening Remarks** *Sylvia Rowe, Food Forum Chair, SR Strategy, LLC, Washington, DC*
9:05 AM	**SESSION 1: What Are Sustainable Diets?** *Session Moderator: Fergus Clydesdale, University of Massachusetts Amherst* **The Dimensions of Sustainability** Adam Drewnowski, University of Washington

Implications and Relevance of Sustainable Diets Internationally: It's All About the Context
Jessica Fanzo, Johns Hopkins University, Food and Agriculture Organization of the United Nations (FAO)

Decision Making Under Uncertainty: Sustainable Diets for Conditions of Scarcity or Abundance
Parke Wilde, Tufts University

30-Minute Moderated Discussion/Q&A

10:35 AM	**15-MINUTE BREAK**
10:50 AM	**SESSION 2: Measurement and Analysis of Sustainable Diets from Production to Consumption** *Session Moderator: Diego Rose, Tulane University*

Mapping Food Supply and Demand: Data Inputs, Metrics, and Measures
Ashkan Afshin, Institute for Health Metrics and Evaluation

Dietary Patterns Link Human Health and the Environment
David Tilman, University of Minnesota

What Makes for Food Systems That Are Sustainable and Resilient?
Mark Rosegrant, International Food Policy Research Institute

20-Minute Moderated Discussion/Q&A

12:10 PM	**LUNCH BREAK**
1:30 PM	**SESSION 3: Sustainability and Healthy Dietary Changes Through Policy and Program Actions** *Session Moderator: David Klurfeld, U.S. Department of Agriculture*

Health and Environmental Benefits of Dietary Changes
Marco Springmann, Oxford University

How to Reduce the Carbon Footprint Without Sacrificing Affordability, Nutrient Density, and Taste
Jennie Macdiarmid, University of Aberdeen (via Zoom)

A Menu of Solutions for a Sustainable Food Future
Janet Ranganathan, World Resources Institute

2:30 PM **20-MINUTE BREAK**

2:50 PM **SESSION 3 Continued**

How to Include Nutrition in All Aspects of the Value Chain
Maha Tahiri, Former Food Industry Executive

Opportunities for Integrating Sustainability and Dietary Guidance
Barbara O. Schneeman, University of California, Davis (Professor Emerita)

30-Minute Moderated Discussion/Q&A

4:00 PM **ADJOURN DAY 1**

DAY 2, AUGUST 2, 9:15 AM–12:00 PM

9:15 AM **Welcome and Opening Remarks**
Sylvia Rowe, Food Forum Chair, SR Strategy, LLC, Washington, DC

9:20 AM **SESSION 4: Innovations in Food Production and Distribution to Reduce Environmental Footprint**
Session Moderator: Kate Houston, Cargill, Inc.

Reducing the Footprint of Animal Agriculture
Frank Mitloehner, University of California, Davis

Reducing the Footprint Through Alternative Diets
Marty Heller, University of Michigan

Local and Regional Food Systems in Sustainable Diets
Nicole Tichenor Blackstone, Tufts University

Retail/Sustainability Across Supply Chain
Karrie Denniston, Walmart

20-Minute Moderated Discussion/Q&A

11:00 AM **Concluding Discussion**
Moderator: Erik Olson, Natural Resources Defense Council

Panelists:

- Connie Avramis, Unilever
- Adam Drewnowski, University of Washington
- Jessica Fanzo, Johns Hopkins University, United Nations FAO
- Diego Rose, Tulane University
- Marco Springmann, Oxford University
- David Tilman, University of Minnesota

12:00 PM **ADJOURN WORKSHOP**

ABOUT US

The Food Forum convenes scientists, administrators, and policy makers from academia, government, industry, and public sectors on an ongoing basis to discuss problems and issues related to food, food safety, and regulation and to identify possible approaches for addressing those problems and issues. The Forum provides a rapid way to identify areas of concordance among these diverse interest groups. It does not make recommendations, nor does it offer specific advice. It does compile information, develop options, and bring interested parties together.

The Food and Nutrition Board (FNB) established the Food Forum in 1993 to allow selected science and technology leaders in the food industry, top administrators in the federal government, representatives from consumer interest groups, and academicians to periodically discuss and debate food and food related issues openly and in a neutral setting. The Forum provides a mechanism for these diverse groups to identify possible approaches for addressing food and food safety problems and issues surrounding the often complex interactions among industry, academia, regulatory agencies, and consumers.

About the FNB: The FNB falls within the Health and Medicine Division of the National Academies of Sciences, Engineering, and Medicine. The National Academies are private, nonprofit institutions that provide independent, objective analysis and advice to the nation to solve complex problems and inform public policy decisions related to science, technology, and medicine. The National Academies operate under an 1863 congressional charter to the National Academy of Sciences, signed by President Lincoln.

http://www.nationalacademies.org/foodforum

B

Acronyms and Abbreviations

CGIAR	Consultative Group on International Agricultural Research
CICERO	Center for International Climate Research
CIW	Coalition of Immokalee Workers
CO_2	carbon dioxide
dataFIELD	database of Food Impacts on the Environment for Linking to Diets
DGA	*Dietary Guidelines for Americans*
DGAC	Dietary Guidelines Advisory Committee
DGPCG	Dietary Guidelines Planning and Continuity Group
DGSAC	Dietary Guidelines Scientific Advisory Committee
EBT	electronic benefits transfer
EFSA	European Food Safety Authority
ENSO	El Niño Southern Oscillation
EPA	U.S. Environmental Protection Agency
eq	equivalent
FAO	Food and Agriculture Organization
FINI	Food Insecurity Nutrition Incentive
FLX	flexitarian diet
FPCM	fat- and protein-corrected milk

GBD	Global Burden of Disease
GDP	gross domestic product
GHG	greenhouse gas
GMO	genetically modified organism
Gt	gigaton
HHS	U.S. Department of Health and Human Services
HIC	high-income country
IFPRI	International Food Policy Research Institute
IFT	Institute of Food Technologists
IHME	Institute for Health Metrics and Evaluation
IMPACT	International Model for Policy Analysis of Agricultural Commodities and Trade
IPCC	Intergovernmental Panel on Climate Change
ISFM	integrated soil fertility management
IUCN	International Union for Conservation of Nature
kcal	kilocalorie
kg	kilogram
LCA	life-cycle analysis
LEAP	Livestock Environmental Assessment and Performance Partnership
LIC	low-income country
LMC	lower-middle-income country
MDG	Millennium Development Goal
N	population
NARS	National Agriculture Research System
NGO	nongovernmental organization
NHANES	National Health and Nutrition Examination Survey
NRF	nutrient-rich food
NSVC	nutrition-sensitive value chain
ODI	Overseas Development Institute
PM	particulate matter
prd	production
PPP	purchasing power parity
PSC	pescetarian diet

SDG	Sustainable Development Goal
SNAP	Supplemental Nutrition Assistance Program
std	standard
TEP	technical expert panel
WHO	World Health Organization
WRI	World Resources Institute
UMC	upper-middle-income country
UN	United Nations
USDA	U.S. Department of Agriculture
VEG	vegetarian diet
VGN	vegan diet

C

Speaker and Moderator Biographies

Ashkan Afshin, Sc.D., M.Sc., M.P.H., M.D., is assistant professor of health metrics sciences at the Institute for Health Metrics and Evaluation (IHME), University of Washington. In this role, he works on the Global Burden of Disease project, leading the effort to estimate the disease burden attributable to dietary risk factors, obesity, and micronutrient deficiencies. Prior to joining IHME, Dr. Afshin completed a postdoctoral fellowship in epidemiology at Tufts University's Friedman School of Nutrition Science and Policy. He was also a postdoctoral fellow at the Harvard T.H. Chan School of Public Health, where he focused on nutrition, chronic disease, and dietary policy. He is a physician and epidemiologist with formal training and experience in health policy, population health, decision sciences, public health informatics, and health economics. Dr. Afshin earned an M.D. from Tehran University of Medical Sciences, an M.P.H. from Johns Hopkins University, and an M.Sc. in health policy and a dual Sc.D. in epidemiology and global health and population from Harvard University.

Connie Avramis, M.Sc., is research and development director, nutrition and health, for Unilever North America. She is responsible for nutrition science, nutrition communications, and health and wellness. In her prior roles, she has held various positions in research and development with global and regional responsibility in both European and developing and emerging markets across retail and food service business units. She is an effective team builder with a proven track record in partnering with brand marketing/sales and the supply chain to translate and develop innovative and differentiating concepts that provide competitive solutions and profitable and sustainable growth.

Nicole Tichenor Blackstone, M.S., Ph.D., is assistant professor in the Division of Agriculture, Food, and Environment at the Friedman School of Nutrition Science and Policy, Tufts University. Prior to joining the Friedman School faculty, she was a postdoctoral research fellow with the Sustainability Institute at the University of New Hampshire. Her research focuses on developing and evaluating strategies for improving food system sustainability. Current and recent research projects include linking sustainability to the *Dietary Guidelines for Americans*, quantifying the environmental and nutritional costs of food waste, developing food waste solutions in the northeastern United States, estimating regional self-reliance and environmental impacts of livestock in the northeastern United States, and developing and assessing core competencies in food systems and sustainability science education. Dr. Blackstone also has experience in food policy spanning the local to national levels through previous work with the Douglas County Food Policy Council (Kansas) and National Family Farm Coalition. She is committed to collaborating across disciplines and with stakeholders to bring about transformative change in the food system. Dr. Blackstone earned her Ph.D. and M.S. from the Friedman School, Tufts University, in the Agriculture, Food, and Environment program. During her graduate training, she was the recipient of multiple fellowships, including the Switzer Environmental Leadership Fellowship. She holds a B.A. in philosophy and religious studies from the University of Kansas.

Fergus "Ferg" Clydesdale, M.A., Ph.D., is currently distinguished university professor, Department of Food Science, University of Massachusetts Amherst, and director of the University of Massachusetts Food Science Policy Alliance. From 1988 to 2008 he was head of the Department of Food Science. His research involves the role of technology in creating healthy and sustainable diets and its regulation and policy. He is a fellow of five premier societies in the field of food science and nutrition, serves as editor-in-chief of *Critical Reviews in Food Science and Nutrition*, and has published some 375 scientific articles and co-authored or edited 20 books. He has held professorships and has given invited presentations around the globe, as well as being an invited speaker in the National Academies series "Distinctive Voices" at the Jonsson Center. Dr. Clydesdale also has served on or chaired numerous committees of various food organizations and agencies, as well as served on the Food and Nutrition Board of the National Academies, the Dietary Guidelines 2005 Scientific Advisory Committee, the Board of Trustees of the International Life Sciences Institute, and the International Food Information Council Foundation. He is the recipient of numerous awards, including the Institute of Food Technologists' highest honor, the Nicolas Appert Award; the University of Massachusetts Amherst Distinguished Teacher Award; and the Distinguished Faculty Award from the University of Massachusetts Alumni Association. He also was named the Sterling B. Hendricks Memorial Lecturer by the Agricultural Research Service/U.S. Department of Agriculture for 2008. The University of Massachusetts Amherst established the Fergus M. Clydesdale Professorship and dedicated the Fergus M. Clydesdale Center for Foods for Health and Wellness in his honor in 2011. Dr. Clydesdale received his M.A. in food chemistry from the University of Toronto and his Ph.D. in food science and technology from the University of Massachusetts Amherst.

Karrie Denniston, M.P.A., serves as senior director of sustainability with the Walmart Foundation. In this role, she manages strategy and grantmaking for the Walmart Foundation's efforts to help create environmentally and socially sustainable supply chains globally. Her portfolio includes elevating dignity in work through empowerment of workers and driving market access for smallholder farmers; creating more sustainable product chains from production to end of life; and addressing hunger, food safety, and nutrition issues. Prior to joining Walmart, Ms. Denniston served as vice president of national programs at Feeding America, the largest hunger relief organization in the United States. She also worked in public service as a policy analyst at the U.S. Department of Agriculture's Food and Nutrition Service, Child Nutrition Division. Ms. Denniston received a B.A. in international relations from the State University of New York at Geneseo and a master's degree in public administration from George Mason University, focused on nonprofit management.

Adam Drewnowski, M.A., Ph.D., is professor of epidemiology and director of the Nutritional Sciences Program at the School of Public Health, University of Washington. He is a world-renowned leader in the study of obesity and social disparities in diets and health. He is also director of the University of Washington Center for Obesity Research, which addresses the environmental, social, and economic aspects of the obesity epidemic. Dr. Drewnowski is adjunct professor of medicine and is a joint member of the Fred Hutchinson Cancer Research Center in Seattle. He is the inventor of the Nutrient Rich Foods Index, which rates individual foods based on their overall nutritional value, and the Affordable Nutrition Index, which helps consumers identify affordable healthy foods. He has conducted extensive studies on taste function and food preferences, exploring the role of fat, sugar, and salt in food preferences and food cravings. His studies on bitter taste genetics have explored consumer acceptance of bitter phytochemicals in vegetables and fruit. Dr. Drewnowski has been the leader in studies of the spatial epidemiology of diets and health, using innovative geographic information systems approaches to study the geographic distribution of food spending, diet quality, and obesity rates. His interests are in characterization of dietary patterns; nutrition economics; the spatial distribution of obesity rates; and the development of new metrics for identifying foods that are nutrient dense, affordable, and sustainable. Dr. Drewnowski obtained his M.A. in biochemistry at Balliol College, Oxford, and a Ph.D. in psychology at The Rockefeller University in New York.

Jessica Fanzo, Ph.D., is Bloomberg distinguished associate professor of global food and agricultural policy and ethics at the Nitze School of Advanced International Studies, the Berman Institute of Bioethics, and the Bloomberg School of Public Health at Johns Hopkins University. She also serves as director of the Global Food Ethics and Policy Program at Hopkins, and plays key advisory roles in Hopkins' Alliance for a Healthier World on the food security and nutrition theme, as well as the Bloomberg American Health Initiative on obesity and food systems. She is currently serving as co-chair for the Global Nutrition Report, and is team leader for the High-Level Panel of Experts for Food Systems and Nutrition for the United Nations Committee on Food Security. She also serves on the *Lancet* Commission on Healthy Diets for Sustainable Food Systems. With more than 15 years of research and program experience working in the field in sub-Saharan Africa and South and East Asia, her expertise focuses on multisectoral and system approaches to ensuring better nutrition and diets, concentrated in three areas: (1) the linkages among agriculture, the environment and climate, and health to improve food systems and environments, diversity and quality of diets, and nutrition outcomes; (2) the importance of regaining food security and agriculture-based livelihoods in postconflict regions through better governance and food policy; and (3) the emerging area of equitable, ethical, and sustainable diets and food systems. Dr. Fanzo was the first laureate of the Carasso Foundation's Sustainable Diets Prize in 2012 for her research on sustainable food and diets for long-term human health. She holds a Ph.D. in nutrition from the University of Arizona and completed a Stephen I. Morse postdoctoral fellowship in immunology in the Department of Molecular Medicine at Columbia University.

Martin Heller, Ph.D., is senior research specialist with the Center for Sustainable Systems at the University of Michigan. His most recent research interests involve evaluating the environmental impact of dietary choices and food waste, and combining nutritional information with environmental assessments of food and diet. A Wellcome Trust–sponsored project in collaboration with nutritionists at Tulane University has provided the first linkage between food-related environmental impacts and National Health and Nutrition Examination Survey datasets. Dr. Heller has conducted life-cycle assessment studies of short-rotation woody biomass energy crops; a plant-based meat alternative "burger"; a large-scale vertically integrated U.S. organic dairy industry; and as part of an international team, a comprehensive, spatially explicit study of U.S. dairy production. He also developed a seminal report on life-cycle-based sustainability indicators for assessment of the U.S. food system. Dr. Heller currently serves on the Menus of Change Scientific and Technical Advisory Council and has been an invited speaker at multiple National Academies workshops on sustainable diets and the true costs of food. He received a B.S. in chemical engineering from Michigan State and a Ph.D., also in chemical engineering, from the University of Colorado Boulder.

Kate J. Houston, M.S., is director, federal government relations/corporate affairs, Cargill, Inc., a global producer and marketer of food, agricultural, financial, and industrial products and services based in Wayzata, Minnesota. Ms. Houston advises Cargill's food and ingredient businesses on critical issues in food safety and nutrition—two public health imperatives important to Cargill's long-term success. She also served as deputy under secretary for the U.S. Department of Agriculture's Food, Nutrition, and Consumer Services mission area, and as a policy advisor to the House of Representatives' Education and the Workforce Committee under the leadership of John A. Boehner, where she worked to enact bipartisan legislation reauthorizing the Child Nutrition and Special Supplemental Nutrition Program for Women, Infants, and Children programs; Head Start; and the Older Americans Act. She holds degrees from Tulane University and the Friedman School of Nutrition Science and Policy at Tufts University, and is a board member of the Congressional Hunger Center; the International Food Information Council; and Common Threads DC, a nonprofit organization preventing obesity by teaching low-income children to cook healthy meals. She received a B.A. in political science and communication from Tulane University and an M.S. in U.S. nutrition policy and epidemiology.

David Klurfeld, M.S., Ph.D., has been national program leader for human nutrition in the U.S. Department of Agriculture's (USDA's) Agricultural Research Service since 2004. He is responsible for the scientific direction of the intramural human nutrition research conducted by USDA laboratories. Prior to government service, he was professor and chairman of the Department of Nutrition and Food Science at Wayne State University in Detroit, Michigan, for 12 years. Before that, he was on the faculty of The Wistar Institute and the University of Pennsylvania School of Medicine for 15 years. His research has focused on the relationship of diet to prevention of chronic diseases such as cancer, heart disease, and gallstones. Among his scientific discoveries are the first demonstration that consumption of red wine results in fewer cardiovascular lesions, that the cholesterol-filled cells in human arterial lesions are white blood cells, that reducing calories is more important than reducing fat in the diet for decreasing cancer growth, and that a mediator of this last effect was likely IGF-1. Dr. Klurfeld has published more than 195 peer-reviewed articles and book chapters. He has been associate editor of the *American Journal for Clinical Nutrition* for 11 years and is also a member of the National Diabetes & Digestive & Kidney Diseases Advisory Council. He is an elected fellow of the American Society for Nutrition. Dr. Klurfeld received his undergraduate degree in general agriculture from Cornell University and both master's and doctorate degrees in pathology from the Medical College of Virginia.

Jennie Macdiarmid, Ph.D., is professor of sustainable nutrition and health at the University of Aberdeen. Her current research focuses on food and nutrition security and the impact of dietary patterns on climate change, in particular understanding how to shift dietary intakes to those that are healthier, more environmentally sustainable, and acceptable to the population. She leads a large multidisciplinary research team, with international collaborations, to address important questions in food and nutrition security. She worked as a research assistant at the Institute of Food Research (Norwich) and the University of Dundee on research focused on eating behaviors, related in particular to chocolate. She spent 18 months working for the International Obesity Task Force, based at the Rowett Research Institute in Aberdeen. In 1999, she moved to the University of Aberdeen Medical School to run a project studying the long-term health effects of professional diving. In 2006, she joined the Public Health Nutrition Research group at the Rowett Institute of Nutrition and Health at the University of Aberdeen, where she is currently a senior research fellow. Professor Macdiarmid graduated from the University of Surrey with a B.Sc. (Hons) in nutrition and food science, and completed her Ph.D. at the University of Leeds on the characteristics of high and low fat consumers.

Frank Mitloehner, M.S., Ph.D., is professor and air quality specialist in cooperative extension in the Department of Animal Science, University of California, Davis. He is an expert in agricultural air quality, livestock housing, and husbandry. Overall, he conducts research that is directly relevant to the understanding and mitigation of air emissions from livestock operations, as well as the implications of these emissions for the health and safety of farm workers and neighboring communities. Dr. Mitloehner has served as chairman of a global United Nations Food and Agriculture Organization partnership project to benchmark the environmental footprint of livestock production. He served as a workgroup member on the President's Council of Advisors on Science and Technology and as a member of the National Academies' Committee on a Framework for Assessing the Health, Environmental, and Social Effects of the Food System. He received his M.S. in animal science and agricultural engineering from the University of Leipzig, Germany, and his Ph.D. in animal science from Texas Technical University.

Erik D. Olson, J.D., is senior strategic director for health and food at the Natural Resources Defense Council. He has more than 25 years of experience in consumer, public health, and environmental policy and advocacy. Prior to joining the Natural Resources Defense Council, he was director of food programs at the Pew Health Group, where he oversaw food-related projects, including programs aimed at improving food safety, strengthening safety and nutrition standards for foods served in the nation's schools, and reviewing the adequacy of the U.S. Food and Drug Administration's programs regulating chemicals added to food. Prior to joining Pew, he was deputy staff director and general counsel for the Senate Committee on Environment and Public Works until November 2008. During his Senate tenure, he worked on environmental issues and on health threats from toxic chemicals, playing a key role in major legislation and hearings on global warming, toxic chemicals, children's environmental health, clean air, drinking water, clean water, and environmental justice, among other issues. He also helped negotiate the key provisions enacted in the Consumer Product Safety Improvement Act of 2008 and the green buildings and green schools provisions of the Energy Independent Security Act of 2007. He received a J.D. from the University of Virginia School of Law.

Janet Ranganathan, M.Sc., is vice president for science and research at the World Resources Institute (WRI), a global research organization that works at the intersection of environment and development in more than 50 countries. She works to strengthen the impact of research and data across WRI's six global programs: Food, Forest, Water, Climate, Energy, and Cities. She plays a lead role supporting WRI Brazil, WRI's sustainable investment project, and WRI's open data platforms. During her tenure, she has held diverse positions across WRI's programs and rolled out numerous initiatives, including Resource Watch, Better Buying Lab, and Creating a Sustainable Food Future. Ms. Ranganathan also founded the Greenhouse Gas Protocol Initiative, an international multistakeholder partnership convened by WRI and the World Business Council for Sustainable Development to develop international greenhouse gas accounting and reporting standards. The Greenhouse Gas Protocol Corporate Standard is now the international accounting and reporting standard for business. Ms. Ranganathan received her master's degree in environmental technology from Imperial College London.

Diego Rose, M.P.H., Ph.D., is professor and director of nutrition at Tulane University's School of Public Health and Tropical Medicine. His research explores the social and economic side of nutrition problems, with a focus on nutrition assistance programs, food security, the food environment, and the environmental impacts of dietary choices. He has studied disparities in access to healthy food and has developed a framework for how the neighborhood retail food environment influences dietary choices and obesity. His current research examines the environmental and health consequences of individual self-selected diets in the United States and the effects of simulated dietary changes on these outcomes. Dr. Rose has served on various panels at the National Academies related to food security and public health, and as a consultant to the United Nations Food and Agriculture Organization and the World Food Programme. He teaches graduate courses in nutrition assessment and food and nutrition policy. Prior to joining the faculty at Tulane, he worked for the U.S. Department of Agriculture's Economic Research Service on domestic food assistance policy and in Mozambique and South Africa on food security and nutrition. He began his nutrition career as the director of a local agency Special Supplemental Nutrition Program for Women, Infants, and Children in a farmworker clinic in rural California. Dr. Rose received his B.S. in nutritional sciences, M.P.H. in public health nutrition, and Ph.D. in agricultural economics from the University of California, Berkeley.

Mark W. Rosegrant, Ph.D., is research fellow emeritus at the International Food Policy Research Institute. He has extensive experience in research and policy analysis in agriculture and economic development and the future of world food security, with an emphasis on water resources and other critical natural resource and agricultural policy issues as they impact food security, rural livelihoods, and environmental sustainability. He is the author or editor of 15 books and more than 100 refereed papers in agricultural economics, water resources, and food policy analysis. Dr. Rosegrant has won numerous awards and is a fellow of the American Association for the Advancement of Science. He is also a fellow of the Agricultural and Applied Economics Association. He received a Ph.D. in public policy from the University of Michigan.

Barbara O. Schneeman, Ph.D., is emeritus professor of nutrition at the University of California, Davis (UCD). From 2004 to 2013, she served as director of the Office of Nutrition, Labeling, and Dietary Supplements at the U.S. Food and Drug Administration. In that position, she oversaw the development of policy and regulations for dietary supplements, labeling, food standards, infant formula, and medical foods and served as U.S delegate to two Codex committees (Food Labeling and Nutrition and Foods for Special Dietary Uses). Prior to 2004, she was a faculty member at UCD in the Food Science and Nutrition departments; she also served in several administrative roles, including dean of the College of Agricultural and Environmental Sciences. Her professional activities include serving as higher education coordinator for the U.S. Agency for International Development on dietary guidelines advisory committees and on the International Life Sciences Institute board as a public trustee, as well as on committees for the National Academy of Sciences, the U.S. Department of Agriculture, the Food and Agriculture Organization, and the World Health Organization. Dr. Schneeman's professional honors include awards from the Institute of Food Technologists; she is also a fellow of the American Society of Nutrition and of the American Association for the Advancement of Science. She is recognized for her work on dietary fiber, gastrointestinal function, the development and use of food-based dietary guidelines, and policy development in food and nutrition. Her education and training include a B.S. in food science from UCD; a Ph.D. in nutrition from the University of California, Berkeley; and a National Institutes of Health postdoctoral fellowship.

Marco Springmann, M.Sc., M.S., Ph.D., is senior researcher in the Centre on Population Approaches for Non-Communicable Disease Prevention in the Nuffield Department of Population Health, and leads the Centre's program on environmental sustainability and public health. He is interested in the health, environmental, and economic dimensions of global food systems. He often uses systems models to provide quantitative estimates on food-related questions. Dr. Springmann joined the Centre in December 2013. Between 2013 and 2017, he was a James Martin fellow of the Oxford Martin Programme on the Future of Food, working with researchers from the Nuffield Department of Population Health, the Department of International Development, and the Environmental Change Institute to develop an integrated model of environmental sustainability, health, and economic development. Since 2017, he has been working on extending the health and environmental aspects of that model as part of the Wellcome Trust–funded project Livestock, Environment and People, working closely with different departments across Oxford as well as with international collaborators. He maintains international research collaborations and has conducted regular placements, including at the International Food Policy Research Institute (United States), Deakin University (Australia), Tsinghua University (China), the Massachusetts Institute of Technology (United States), Resources for the Future (United States), the European Investment Bank (Luxembourg), and the German Federal Ministry for the Environment (Germany). He is a junior research fellow at Linacre College and an honorary research associate in the Food Systems Group of the Environmental Change Institute. Dr. Springmann holds a Ph.D. in economics from the University of Oldenburg

(Germany), an M.Sc. in sustainability from the University of Leeds (United Kingdom), and an M.S. in physics from Stony Brook University (United States).

Maha Tahiri, Ph.D., is adjunct professor at the Friedman School of Nutrition Science and Policy at Tufts University. Previously, she served as vice president, chief health and wellness officer at General Mills, Inc., for more than 6 years. She also headed the Bell Institute of Health and Nutrition, which integrates nutrition science, regulatory expertise, and communications to deliver strategic innovation in health and nutrition for all General Mills businesses globally. Her 20-year career spans roles at the intersection of scientific research, innovation, and health communication in multiple food categories and companies covering several regions, including Europe, Asia, the Middle East, and North Africa. Dr. Tahiri serves on the advisory council on nutrition and food choices at the Foundation of Food and Agricultural Research. She is a trustee of the International Food Information Council (IFIC) Foundation. She also serves on the Strategic Oversight Committee of the American Society of Nutrition. In her current and previous leadership roles, she has held several board and scientific advisory board positions in International Life Science Institute branches, IFIC, and the European Food Information Council. Dr. Tahiri is active in developing partnerships across industry, academia, government, and nongovernmental organizations to tackle complex issues related to nutrition and health.

David Tilman, Ph.D., is Regents' professor and McKnight presidential chair in ecology at the University of Minnesota, where he also serves as director of the Cedar Creek Ecosystem Science Reserve. He is best known for his experimental and theoretical work on competition and on the mechanistic causes of multispecies coexistence, and for demonstrating via rigorous field experiments and theory that biodiversity is of central importance to the functioning of ecosystems. A major goal of his current research is the pursuit of ways to preserve the world's biodiversity, slow the rate of climate change, and still meet human needs for food and energy. He is a member of the National Academy of Sciences and the American Academy of Arts and Sciences, and a foreign member of The Royal Society (London). He was awarded the International Prize for Biology in 2008, the Heineken Prize for Environmental Sciences in 2010, the Balzan Prize in 2014, and the BBVA Foundation's Frontiers of Knowledge Award in 2015. He has received the Cooper and MacArthur Awards from the Ecological Society of America, the Centennial Award from the Botanical Society of America, and a Guggenheim Fellowship, and was named an honorary member or fellow of both the British Ecological Society and the Ecological Society of America. Dr. Tilman received his Ph.D. in zoology from the University of Michigan in 1976.

Parke E. Wilde, Ph.D., is professor at the Friedman School of Nutrition Science and Policy, Tufts University. He conducts research on topics in U.S. food and nutrition policy, including federal food assistance programs and the geography of local food retail. He authored the textbook *Food Policy in the United States: An Introduction* (Routledge, 2018), now in its second edition. Dr. Wilde was a member of the National Academies' Food Forum from 2011 to 2014, and served on the planning committee for a workshop on Sustainable Diets: Food for Healthy People and a Healthy Planet (2013). He holds a B.A. in political science from Swarthmore College and an M.S. and a Ph.D. in agricultural economics from Cornell University.